In the Shadow of the Eighth

In the Shadow of the Eighth

the Eighth

My Forty Years Working for Women's

Health in Ireland

PETER BOYLAN

PENGUIN

IRELAND

For Jane

PENGUIN IRELAND

UK | USA | Canada | Ireland | Australia
India | New Zealand | South Africa

Penguin Ireland is part of the Penguin Random House group of companies
whose addresses can be found at global.penguinrandomhouse.com.

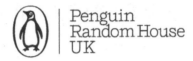

First published 2019
001

Copyright © Peter Boylan, 2019

The moral right of the author has been asserted

Set in 12/14.75 pt Bembo Book MT Std
Typeset by Jouve (UK), Milton Keynes
Printed and bound in Great Britain by Clays Ltd, Elcograf S.p.A.

A CIP catalogue record for this book is available from the British Library

ISBN: 978-1-844-88482-7

MIX
Paper from
responsible sources
FSC
www.fsc.org   FSC® C018179

Penguin Random House is committed to a
sustainable future for our business, our readers
and our planet. This book is made from Forest
Stewardship Council® certified paper.

Contents

PART I

1.   A lucky start in life

In 1973, when I was a student doctor doing the required eight-week obstetrics rotation at Holles Street, the hospital had three antenatal wards, each with around twenty beds. One of these wards was solely for women who were known as 'inuptas', from the Latin for 'unmarried'; at the time almost a quarter of all births to unmarried mothers in the Republic of Ireland took place in Holles Street. The majority of these women came in from Mother and Baby Homes to have their babies. I recall mention of homes in Eglinton Road and Dunboyne, and some of them must also have come from Magdalene Laundries.

As my career progressed, and as I grew as a person and as a doctor, I came to question why we treated women this way. But as a young doctor in training I did not wonder about the effective segregation of these women in the National Maternity Hospital, and neither did anyone else; unconsciously, most of us had absorbed the norms of the time. I might have thought I was worldly, but, as a young man who came from a solidly middle-class Dublin background, I had had no exposure to a side of Irish life that was harsh, judgemental and punitive.

I was born on 7 July 1950, the youngest of four children, following Hugo, Anna and Kate. I did not thrive in my first few weeks – I would vomit my feed up to several feet away, a dramatic and alarming symptom known as projectile vomiting. This led to dehydration and malnutrition, and at six weeks old I was dangerously ill. My mother, who had trained as a nurse and was not inclined to kowtow to doctors, or indeed anyone else, did not feel that our GP was taking the matter seriously enough. She phoned Colman Saunders, a consultant paediatrician, and described my symptoms. He immediately diagnosed pyloric stenosis, a condition present from birth, caused by blockage of the stomach by an overgrowth of muscle. He referred me urgently to John Shanley, the first specialist paediatric surgeon in Ireland, who operated successfully.

As a young schoolboy, when I felt like a day off, I used my infant surgery to my advantage, saying that I had a pain in my tummy

around the scar. I would be allowed to stay at home for the day, rest-
ing in bed, as my mother brought me orange juice and the *Dandy* and
Beano comics. Of course, she knew perfectly well that I was playing
up, but, as the youngest of her children, and the one who had nearly
died, I was somewhat indulged.

My mother, Patricia Clancy, was born in 1913, in Coalisland, County
Tyrone, the tenth of twelve children. After school she followed her
elder sister Mena to Leeds General Infirmary, now St James's University Hospital, where she spent four years training. In 1937 she persuaded
her retired parents to move from Belfast to Dublin, and that same year
she auditioned successfully for the Abbey School of Acting. For over
twenty-five years she was a regular on Austin Clarke's Monday-
evening programmes of poetry readings on Radio Éireann.

My father, Henry – always Harry in the family – was a civil ser-
vant, at that time in the Land Commission, and he took the train
most mornings from our home in Dundrum to Harcourt Street, usually managing a game of poker on the short journey with four other
young men, regular commuters.

My parents had married in 1941, my father having fallen in love
with my mother's voice, speaking verse on Radio Éireann, and
declaring that he 'must meet the owner of that voice'. And in his
determined way he did. As children, we would gather round the
radio with my father and listen to her disembodied voice – a great
source of wonder. I have a clear memory of lying on a rug, peering at
the radio, which was on the floor, listening to my mother reading
poetry, and wondering how on earth she was able to make herself so
small as to fit inside the radio.

My father came from a long line of mariners, going back at least to
the mid 1700s. There is a graveyard at Mornington at the mouth of
the River Boyne where headstones record the lives of numerous Boylan seafarers. Among them is a Captain Peter Boylan, born in 1833,
the son and grandson of pilots of Drogheda harbour and port who
owned a 65-ton pilot boat called *Gazelle*. My great-grandfather Captain William Boylan sailed his own 84-ton schooner called *The Eagle*,
along the coast of France and Spain, into the Mediterranean and
through the Sea of Marmara as far as Constantinople (now Istanbul),
bringing cargos of linen from the nearby mills and returning with
spices and silks from the East. In 1879 he slipped and fell while

boarding his ship in Bordeaux. He had died by the time the ship docked in Drogheda. It was the end of the Boylan shipping line, but not the end of the family love of seafaring.

My grandfather Captain John Boylan followed in the family tradition and went to sea at sixteen, but, as there was no family schooner for him to take over, he shipped in Liverpool on the *Dun Cow*, a three-masted tea-clipper that he went on to captain, and that journeyed on trading routes from Drogheda, around Cape Horn, to San Francisco and back. As my father recalled in his memoir, *A Voyage around My Life*, those were 'the days of wooden ships and iron men . . . [when] . . . one had to be strong, active, hardy and fearless'.

On leaving school, my father, too, would have gone to sea, like two of his elder brothers, but the Great Depression and the collapse of international trade and shipping meant that there were no opportunities for a newcomer. There was no money for university, and he did not want to join a bank or insurance company. Nor did he want to teach ('I did not want to be a National Teacher under the jurisdiction of a parish priest,' he wrote later). Instead he sat the highly competitive civil service exams and joined the Land Commission. The sea was in his blood, however, as it is in mine. He taught me to sail at the age of seven and I have been enjoying it ever since.

I started school in Ardtona House, a small school run by Judy Rogerson in her family home on Lower Churchtown Road. The school is still there. At seven I moved to St Mary's College in Rathmines, chosen largely because my father had been in school with the then head of the College, Fr Paddy Murray, and so the decision was an easy one. By this time we were living in Orwell Park in Rathgar, and I took the No. 14 bus to school every day from the end of the road.

I enjoyed my time at St Mary's enormously, playing countless games of rugby in the winter, and cricket, tennis and basketball in the summer. Towards the end of junior school my academic performance began to slip significantly, and my father threatened to send me to board at Rockwell College in County Tipperary if I didn't pull my socks up. This did not appeal at all. I had run away from Cub camp, hating the discomforts of camping compared to the comforts of home, and did not intend to repeat the experience. The threat of Rockwell worked like a dream. Within two terms I had progressed sufficiently to be transferred from the B class into the A stream.

Rugby was central to my life. I won a Leinster Schools Senior Cup Medal in 1965, while still in fourth year. The next year we were beaten by Blackrock College in the final. In 1967 I was captain, and hoped to lead a successful campaign. Disastrously, however, we were beaten in the first round by Gonzaga – not then known for success in rugby – in a sudden-death play-off, having drawn with them twice. Friends who went to Gonzaga, and others, never tire of reminding me of that defeat, more than fifty years later. Character-building stuff. I played for Leinster Schools in fifth and sixth year, and Leinster under-19s and 21s while in college.

My long-suffering mother used to dread my return from matches. Would I have a black eye, be on crutches or only bruised? In those days, of course, parents seldom went to school rugby games. Perhaps the most spectacular injury was when I almost bisected my tongue in a Leinster Schools trial match in Donnybrook. There was blood everywhere. I was brought to the old St Vincent's casualty department in St Stephen's Green, where the casualty officer inserted stitches into my tongue, without anaesthetic, to hold it together. The upside of this was that I was unable to answer questions in school for weeks afterwards.

My bedroom was at the front of the house in Orwell Park. From the window I watched early-morning activity on the road with particular attention to the cars our neighbours drove. In the 1960s it was the husbands who went to their offices in the mornings. I wondered about their work. My parents may have been literary, interested in the arts, and perhaps holding less conventional views than their neighbours, but Orwell Park was a solidly professional milieu. Our neighbours included two medical consultants, two solicitors, and a stockbroker who lived next door.

The time came when I had to choose a career. In my early teens I wanted to be an actor, a leaning inherited from my mother possibly, but my parents were insistent that I would have to finish school before considering such a precarious existence. With the passage of time the wish to become an actor faded, though I have retained a facility for mimicry and accents. As I progressed through secondary school, I began to consider either law or medicine, both of which appealed. However, law seemed to involve a lot of specialized reading and not much action, whereas medicine was practical. I thought it would suit me best.

At that time to be accepted into pre-med at UCD Medical School, students had to have achieved two honours subjects in the Leaving Certificate. As an insurance policy, to be on the safe side, I took four honours subjects – English, French, Chemistry and Physics – and entered UCD Medical School in October 1968.

At our first Pre-Med lecture in Belfield, we were invited to 'Look at the person sitting on your right – only one of you will be here next year.' I survived the 50 per cent cull at the end of Pre-Med and progressed to First Year Medicine and beyond. I have to admit that I did not achieve honours at any stage, though I won both the Edward A. Smith Medal in obstetrics and the Colman Saunders Medal in paediatrics. Colman Saunders himself presented me with the medal, and I was thrilled to be able to tell him how he had saved my life when I was only six weeks old.

The days in medical school were long, with lectures from 9 to 5, five days a week. With study on top, this left little time for extra-curricular activities. I did, however, manage to play rugby and was captain of the Freshers team in my second year. I played Hospitals Cup rugby every year in college for the St Vincent's team, and we won the cup several times.

In the summer holidays between second and third year of medical school I worked in the Meath Hospital as a porter. My aunt Mena Lambert was a theatre sister there, and she organized the job for me. Looking back, I see how fortunate I was in my connections and contacts. One of my jobs was to bring patients to and from the operating theatre. One day I was wheeling an American woman to theatre on a trolley, and we got talking. I mentioned that I was planning to go to the States the next summer to work in an American hospital. She was from San Francisco and her husband was a successful Irish-American businessman. She asked if I might be interested in going to California. I was, but the problem was that hospitals in California did not pay students because it was so popular that students were happy to work for nothing. 'Leave it with me,' the American patient told me, and from that casual conversation on the way to theatre came a wonderful opportunity: her husband agreed to sponsor me to attend Stanford University Hospital, where he had a physician friend.

So I flew to San Francisco, was given a room in a house in Palo Alto owned by friends of my benefactor, and an American Jeep to drive. Could life be better?

Apparently so. One weekend I was invited to a party in Menlo Park, a wealthy area beside Palo Alto, given by a Mrs Ziski. As I was leaving, she asked me what car I was driving. I explained about the Jeep and she said, 'Oh, but you must have my car for the summer – I'm going to the Far East.' My attempts to decline the offer were rebuffed, and I spent the rest of the summer driving around California in a white Mercedes 250.

It's obvious to me now how lucky I was in my childhood and university days. Three elements emerge as important. My family life was secure and loving. We were all great readers, interested in the arts, discussion and the wider world. Above all my parents were independent thinkers, unafraid to challenge orthodoxies.

Rugby and sailing, meanwhile, taught me the importance of having someone in charge, a captain, who takes responsibility for decisions. Not letting down one's teammates, on or off the pitch, is a feature of team games like rugby, and players who don't understand this pretty soon lose their teammates' regard.

Finally, it is important not to take disagreements personally, to respect one's opponents and to recognize that when the final whistle blows or the finishing line is crossed, hostilities come to an end. These principles have stood to me throughout my professional life.

2. Choosing obstetrics

In 1974 I qualified as a doctor and commenced work in July as an intern at St Vincent's Hospital, which had moved from St Stephen's Green to Elm Park in Merrion four years earlier.

Interns are the lowest rung of the medical ladder, and are assigned to a team or teams led by consultants. We lived in the hospital residence, or 'Res', each of us having our own room, which contained a bed, a desk, wash-hand basin, a wardrobe and little else. Our duties included admitting and discharging patients, reviewing blood results and filing them in the charts, fetching X-rays from the radiology department, sometimes making presentations to the weekly clinical pathological conference, and writing consult cards requesting that a consultant of a different specialty review a patient on the ward.

In the first six months I interned on the surgical side of things. All of the consultants were extremely skilled and very hard-working. Interns will mess when they can, however. For instance, if a patient had a complex medical condition it was often necessary to get a medical consult prior to their having surgery. If the patient had health insurance – and the VHI was then the only option for insurance – one of our number would sometimes ring the letters v h i on the request cards and wait, with a certain amount of cynical amusement, to see if this prompted a quicker response from consultants.

While I enjoyed this time, I concluded that a career in surgery would mean less contact with patients. It is a very technical specialty, and patients' personal histories are almost irrelevant. I prefer interacting with patients.

For my six months on the medical side I worked with Professor Frank Muldowney. He had spent some years in the United States and specialized in metabolic and renal medicine. Metabolic medicine specialists combine a grasp of complex biochemistry with an understanding of the body's metabolism. Renal specialists treat diseases of the kidney. Professor Muldowney had one of the sharpest minds I have ever come across and a great ability to simplify complicated matters.

He had his own laboratory in the department, beside the ward, because he was keen to oversee the quality of biochemical analysis himself and did not want to rely on the general hospital laboratories.

One of our duties as interns was to conduct a daily urine sample analysis of every patient on the ward, primarily to look for any bacterial organisms that might indicate a urinary tract infection, and present the results on ward rounds. In those days, ward rounds were rather like those conducted by the fearsome Sir Lancelot Spratt in *Doctor in the House*. The consultant led his team of research fellows, registrars and senior house officers, with the interns trailing in their august wake.* During rounds, the unfortunate doctor presenting the patient's history would stand facing Professor Muldowney, while we formed a respectful ring behind the great man. On one occasion one of our colleagues, when asked what he had seen looking down the microscope at a patient's urine sample, stuttered over bacterial organisms, reporting that he had seen multiple orgasms. Those of us standing behind Professor Muldowney went into contortions trying to suppress our laughter. We had previously observed that when he was annoyed his ears would go red. On this occasion it looked as if they might catch fire.

On another occasion I was given the task of drawing about twenty blood samples from one of Muldowney's long-term patients who had been admitted for a series of complicated tests. I duly sent them to the laboratory, and the patient was discharged home with an appointment to come to an outpatient clinic for review of the results. To my horror, when the results came back, written across each one was 'Not possible to analyse, blood in wrong tube'. I knew perfectly well what the professor's reaction would be, but my fellow interns came to my rescue. When the patient returned to the clinic, we were all alerted to watch for his file and hide it. He was spirited away into a side room and given another appointment for a few days after our departure, when the new team of interns would have to deal with Muldowney's reaction. (I should add that no harm came to the patient as a consequence of this and indeed he rather enjoyed his time on the ward, but I wouldn't recommend such a course of action to trainees today.)

In the 1970s the Sisters of Charity were actively involved in running St Vincent's. Each ward had a nun in charge and they ran a tight

---

* In those days it was always 'his' – in Irish hospitals, consultants were always men.

ship. I well remember Sr Borgia, known to generations of junior doctors and nurses as 'The Borge', who instilled great fear in us lowly interns. She had a determined manner and the disconcerting habit of calling patients by the number on their beds rather than by their names. She was very severe to her student nurses and doctors, and even the most senior consultants treated her with considerable respect. Sr Borgia was, however, devoted and kind to her patients. She worked a lot at night and, at a time when medication was not as tightly controlled as it is today, she had a ready supply of morphine tablets in her pocket that she dispensed as she saw fit to very elderly, very ill patients, who were not long for the world.

Following our intern year we had to decide what path we would take in our future careers. I didn't need to give it much thought. During my eight weeks' placement at Holles Street as a medical student, the hospital's former master, Kieran O'Driscoll, set all his students a task. We were each to stay with six women having their first babies. And then we were to write an essay on how we viewed their experiences of the labour and birth. Their experiences, not ours. We were to forget about the physical aspects of childbirth. So we weren't to get involved in describing how blood pressure varied, or how much blood the women lost, or how many stitches were required. That wasn't the point. Instead we were told to focus on the new mothers' emotional experience.

Being present there, alongside young women having their first babies – and actually witnessing the births – had a profound influence on me. As a young male medical student, that experience taught me a great deal: to observe just how women cope with the stress and pain of labour, and how, with the birth of a healthy baby, there is such a transformation in their emotions, from extreme stress and anxiety to utter joy. All through my later career I never lost the feeling of what a privilege it was to be present when a woman gave birth.

Having interviewed successfully, I started at Holles Street in July 1975 for a six-month rotation as a senior house officer (SHO) in obstetrics, to be followed by six months each in neonatology and gynaecology.

The work was hard and the hours were long – it was not unusual to be on-duty for twenty-four hours straight. We would be on the go all night looking after women in labour, doing deliveries, assisting with

Caesarean sections. At 11 a.m. every morning there was a coffee break in the doctors' residence. Consultants and juniors mixed together in the Res, and it was an opportunity to learn and discuss difficult cases. The informal gathering allowed the consultants to get to know the junior staff, and it allowed us juniors to observe the consultants in action. The atmosphere between doctors, midwives and other staff was collegial. I knew almost immediately that obstetrics was right for me.

Obstetrics is, generally speaking, a happy and emotionally rewarding specialty. The majority of labours and deliveries are uncomplicated, but occasionally things go suddenly and catastrophically wrong, leading to the death of a baby or, the ultimate tragedy, the death of a mother. Everyone knew that these outcomes were no respecters of reputation, and so there was no room for complacency or a feeling of superiority.

Some telling numbers show the dramatic improvements in obstetric care from when I started back in 1975 to the present day.

In the mid 1970s there were around 7,500 deliveries in Holles Street each year, of which about 35 per cent were to first-time mothers, compared with 45 per cent today.

Only 11 per cent of women were thirty-five years old or more, compared with more than 40 per cent today.

The figure for women who had at least five children already was 10 per cent, whereas now it is under 1 per cent.

In 1975 just under 7,500 babies were born after twenty-eight weeks gestation. Of these, 150 were either still-born or did not survive beyond the first week. This gave a perinatal mortality rate of 19.8 per thousand births. The corresponding figure for 2017 was 4.6 per thousand.

And, of course, there were significant differences in the practice of obstetrics then, compared with today.

Almost no epidurals were administered in 1974, while the current rate of epidural for relief of pain in labour runs at around 70 per cent for women having their first baby and at about 40 per cent for women having their second or subsequent babies.

Virtually all Caesarean sections are now performed under epidural or spinal anaesthesia, whereas when I first started in Holles Street all women had a general anaesthetic.

In 1975 there were 307 Caesarean sections, while in 2016 there were 2,303, a huge increase in numbers as well as in rate, from around 4 per cent to around 27 per cent. Today, for example, almost 100 per cent of babies presenting by the breech are delivered by Caesarean section, whereas in the early 1970s only 25 per cent of breech babies born to first-time mothers, and fewer than 10 per cent of those born to mothers who already had a baby, were delivered by Caesarean section.

For mainly religious reasons, no tubal ligations* were performed in 1974, whereas by 1997, the last year of my mastership, there were 445 tubal ligations. It should be noted that these numbers have diminished considerably to fewer than fifty a year currently, thanks to advances in contraception, and the introduction of the Mirena coil in particular.

The contraceptive pill was about fifteen years old when I was first at Holles Street, but of course its use was not legal in Ireland. At that time it was prescribed as a 'cycle regulator', and Irish women apparently had the highest rate of irregular cycles anywhere in the Western world.

In the mid 1970s treatment for premature newborn infants was limited. In Holles Street there were just two consultant paediatricians on the staff, both of whom were part time, and the non-consultant staff consisted of one registrar and three senior house officers.

By 2016 there were eleven consultant paediatricians, ten specialist registrars and nine senior house officers in the neonatal department.

The master of Holles Street in 1975 was Declan Meagher, a man I admired enormously and from whom I learned a lot. He was hugely skilled and showed great empathy with patients.† During my time as a senior house officer I worked particularly closely with Kieran O'Driscoll, whose teaching had had such an impact on me when I was a student. He was a visionary doctor who revolutionized the care of women in labour. Paradoxically, however, he was later one of the founding members of the Pro Life Amendment Campaign (PLAC).

Following his appointment as master in 1963, O'Driscoll had

---

* Popularly known as having one's 'tubes tied', the tubes being the woman's Fallopian tubes – a permanent method of contraception, as it prevents egg and sperm meeting.
† Declan Meagher later became my father-in-law when his daughter Frances, also a doctor, and I married.

become concerned about the effect of prolonged labours and maternal exhaustion on women in childbirth. In 1963 a prolonged labour
was defined as seventy-two hours or more, and it was not unusual for
labour to go on for days, ending with an exhausted woman being
sedated with chloroform and undergoing a difficult forceps delivery,
often with associated haemorrhage and damage to the birth canal.

O'Driscoll recognized that on a first birth this had potentially
very serious implications, both for a woman's future childbearing –
many women ended up with a feeling of revulsion for childbirth – and
for her bonding with her children and relationship with her husband.
He wanted to make labour a more humane process for the mother
and looked at ways of reducing her exposure to physical and emotional stress.

As he undertook his study of labour, he recognized that there were
fundamental differences between a first birth and subsequent births.
He set about looking at ways of reducing the duration of labour and
developed a series of protocols that became well established in Holles
Street, though not elsewhere in Ireland. O'Driscoll met with some
opposition from mainly older colleagues who were extremely conservative and regarded any change as interference in the natural
process of childbirth.

O'Driscoll's work attracted considerable international attention, particularly after the 1969 publication of a paper titled 'Prevention of
Prolonged Labour' in the *British Medical Journal*. He referred to the management and active involvement of senior clinicians in the care of all
women in labour, not just those with complications. The *British Medical
Journal* wrote an accompanying editorial and used the title 'Active Management of Labour (AML)'. O'Driscoll's approach now had a name.

As O'Driscoll developed AML, he honed it to consist of a series of
minor interventions, including breaking of the waters when they had
not already broken, administration of oxytocin* when a labour was
progressing slowly and, perhaps most importantly of all, assigning
each woman in labour her own individual midwife over the course of

---

* Oxytocin is a hormone that, among other things, helps the process of childbirth.
Synthetic oxytocin supplements a woman's naturally occurring oxytocin. It
increases the force of uterine contractions and is used to accelerate the progress of
labour or to induce a labour that has not started.

that labour (within the constraints of midwifery shift times). His objective was less that the midwife was to monitor the woman's physical status – he recognized that the majority of women having children are healthy and just happen to be pregnant and going through childbirth – but rather to provide emotional support. At that time it was unusual for the husband to be present throughout the labour, although that became more common with the passage of time. (Generally speaking, in those days women went into hospital with husbands; few unmarried women presented with partners, male or female.)

AML was particularly helpful in reducing the incidence of abnormal labour, known as dystocia. Prior to the development of AML, women in prolonged labour, often for more than twenty-four hours, were delivered by Caesarean section, by difficult and traumatic forceps delivery, or by using symphysiotomy to widen the pelvis.* AML reduced the incidence of traumatic forceps deliveries and made symphysiotomy obsolete. O'Driscoll and his successor as master, Declan Meagher, published their work in a manual entitled *Active Management of Labour: The Dublin Experience.*†

Unfortunately, in recent years AML has sometimes been represented as a method of controlling women and interfering with the natural process of childbirth. Despite all the evidence of the benefits to women, one occasionally comes across this misrepresentation. The definition of what constituted prolonged labour decreased progressively with the refinement and development of AML, and by the early 1970s O'Driscoll could show that when AML protocols were followed, fewer than 5 per cent of women had labours lasting more than twelve hours. The benefits, both physical and emotional, to women were enormous.

Obstetricians and midwives today come from all over Europe, especially the Nordic countries, to participate in AML courses at Holles Street twice a year. I continue to teach on this course and emphasize the importance of what I learned in the early years of my

---

* Symphysiotomy is an incision in the joint at the front of the pelvis that allows a widening of the pelvis to facilitate safe vaginal delivery. Its use today is restricted to rare emergencies.

† I was co-author of the revised Third Edition issued in 1993.

career to balance the physical and emotional needs of a woman in labour and to care for her holistically.

Kieran O'Driscoll was a hard taskmaster but had a twinkle in his eye. His humanity also made a lasting impression on me. On one occasion we examined a woman in her early forties, on her first pregnancy after a long history of infertility. She had been admitted for an elective Caesarean section. At that time elective Caesareans were extremely unusual, and O'Driscoll was particularly proud of the hospital's low section rate, at only 4 per cent in 1975. We were therefore curious as to why he wasn't encouraging a vaginal delivery.

'This is not obstetrics', came the reply; 'this woman needs her baby.'

He recognized that it was probably her only chance of having a baby and so no risk was acceptable. This, of course, was in the days long before I V F or any other type of assisted fertility treatment was available. It was, for that time, an unusual example of a consultant listening to the woman.*

O'Driscoll supported me in my early research. I set out to see if I could answer a simple question: did oxytocin cause neonatal jaundice? This was a controversial topic in the medical journals at the time. It had been postulated that neonatal jaundice might be a toxic side effect of synthetic oxytocin. If oxytocin did indeed have a toxic effect on the baby, it would be difficult to justify its continued use in the care of women in labour.

I undertook a study of 200 consecutive first-born infants whose mothers had started labour spontaneously, and my subsequent findings – that the use of oxytocin was not toxic to the baby – were published in the *British Medical Journal* in September 1976. It was my first publication.

Before I submitted it, I had asked O'Driscoll if he would put his name to it, partly because I felt his prestige would add authority to the work and increase its chances of publication, but mainly because

---

* Paradoxically, given his compassion and empathy, he was later one of the founding members of the Pro Life Amendment Campaign, as mentioned above. He was not unique. Over the course of my career I met other good and caring doctors who had an absolutist anti-abortion mind-set. Given what they knew about pregnancy, and about women's lives, I found that mind-set hard to fathom. Catholic teaching undoubtedly influenced many of them, including O'Driscoll.

he had been so encouraging. He declined. I had done all the work, he said, and he would not take any credit. The *BMJ* published it anyway. It was an interesting example of Kieran O'Driscoll's integrity. Those of us in medical circles (and probably other fields) know academics whose names appear as co-authors on papers where junior staff have in fact done all the work.

After my six months in obstetrics I worked for six months as an SHO in the neonatal department, and my final six months in the NMH were spent as senior house officer in gynaecology, giving me an opportunity to learn the fundamentals of gynaecological surgery. Because I had been in the hospital for a year at that stage I was encouraged to accept more responsibilities when on-duty. The two assistant masters at the time, Carthage Carroll and Malachy Coughlan, encouraged me and were wonderful colleagues in terms of training and support. By the time my rotation finished, I was confident in performing Caesarean sections and minor gynaecological procedures. And then it was time to gain more experience. I needed to leave Holles Street behind me for a time. But I vowed I would be back. I knew then I wanted to spend my professional life in the place where I felt really at home.

3.   A new perspective on abortion

In December 1976 I moved to London to a six-month position at Queen Charlotte's Maternity Hospital in Chiswick, one of the oldest maternity hospitals in Europe.* I lived in a flat nearby owned by the hospital. My flatmate was an anaesthetist who had fled Czechoslovakia, leaving behind his wife and young child. He had hoped to be able to smuggle them to England but was unsuccessful, and he missed them terribly. He spent much of his spare time in his room listening to the BBC World Service, keeping up to date with events behind the Iron Curtain. It was an education for me about the inhumane consequences of the Communist regimes of Eastern Europe and a broadening of my horizons.

Queen Charlotte's had a very good reputation in the obstetric world, and a lot of research was conducted there. However, the practice of obstetrics was very different from what I was used to. I had become accustomed to AML, to midwives taking the lead in a delivery, and being instructed by the senior midwife regarding the care of the woman in labour. She (and it was always a 'she' in the 1970s) would decide, for example, when an operative vaginal delivery – forceps, perhaps – was necessary, and we would be summoned to perform the delivery (under her eagle eye). This made sense – we were callow junior doctors and the senior midwives had years of experience. In Queen Charlotte's, however, women were not assigned an individual midwife and junior doctors were expected to make all the decisions.

Another difference demonstrated the benefits of AML. A particular type of forceps, known as Kielland's, used to rotate the baby's head when it was in the wrong position, had been abandoned in Holles Street in the late 1960s. At Queen Charlotte's, however, Kielland's forceps were deployed on a regular basis. A disturbing case illustrated graphically to me why these particular forceps were no longer in use in Holles Street. On one occasion a colleague used them

* Queen Charlotte's was founded in 1739.

on a woman in order to effect delivery, but in the process she unfortunately experienced a very large spiral tear in the vagina that extended up into the cervix and uterus, and the baby was still-born. Autopsy of the baby showed an intracranial haemorrhage that was traumatic in origin as a consequence of the use of the forceps. The mother underwent emergency surgery and was advised that she should not become pregnant again. It was her first child.

One of the reasons why the Kielland's forceps had been abandoned in the NMH was because AML had made their use superfluous. Increasing the strength of the contractions with oxytocin helped the baby's head rotate as it passed through the birth canal, thereby making it unnecessary to rotate it in any other way. This was a medical solution to a problem that was treated surgically, with forceps, elsewhere.

After six months I was lucky to be selected to continue my training at the Chelsea Hospital for Women for a year. The Chelsea Hospital for Women was a distinctly British institution, with characteristics suggestive of the army or a public school. There was a dining room for consultants and junior doctors, for example, where lunch was served from large silver dishes on a sideboard.

Head of the service at the Chelsea Hospital was Professor Jack Dewhurst, who was internationally recognized for his work in paediatric and adolescent gynaecology and intersex conditions. Though he was a practising Roman Catholic, he was also president of the Royal College of Obstetricians and Gynaecologists, which had a liberal attitude towards abortion. He was a pragmatic and consensual president who steered the College through many of the ethical controversies of the 1970s, such as the in-vitro fertilization debate, which happened on his watch. Seeing how Jack Dewhurst conducted himself was enlightening: I could see that someone could hold a particular belief – in his case religious – while at the same time respecting the very different beliefs of others.

When I finished my clinical post at the Chelsea in July 1978, I spent two years as a research fellow at Queen Charlotte's and the Hammersmith hospitals. I undertook a research project that looked at fetal behaviour in labour, which involved recruiting women in the antenatal clinic in order to study fetal breathing movements both before and during labour. Babies don't actually breathe while in the womb, but for about 35 per cent of the time before labour starts they make movements that mimic breathing. Recent research from Oxford had suggested that fetal breathing movements continued during labour but were suppressed if the baby was beginning to experience a lack of oxygen.

I attempted to replicate this work using more sophisticated equipment than had been available to the Oxford researchers. I compared the number of fetal breathing movements antenatally and during labour in twenty-two women, and my conclusion was that the cessation of fetal breathing movements in labour was normal, but that the cause of this change in behaviour had not been positively identified. In other words, it wasn't indicative of fetal distress. This work directly contradicted the conclusions of the Oxford group but came to be the accepted science. (Subsequent research suggested that it was a hormone, prostaglandin, that suppressed fetal breathing movements in labour.)

Another arm of my research was to study the effect of alcohol on fetal breathing movements, which are a reflection of central nervous system activity. This original research work was the basis of the thesis for my Master in the Art of Obstetrics (MAO) Degree from University College Dublin, which I was awarded in 1983.

The great advantage of my research post in London was that I was not rostered for duty at either Queen Charlotte's or the Chelsea for the duration, and so my working hours were more regular than they had been for years. I had joined London Irish Rugby Football Club when I arrived in London and was now able to spend more time playing rugby. The club had a fantastic mix of players from all backgrounds: professionals from the North and South of Ireland and from the UK, farmers, builders, labourers and sons of Irish immigrants. We were a very broad church and I made many friends. Members of the team were playing international rugby also. Doctors Ken Kennedy and John O'Driscoll toured with the British and Irish Lions, and it was a great honour to play regularly with such legends.

Another doctor, Pat Parfrey from Cork, was the captain of London Irish when I was there. He was a tough coach, with both a strong personality and a strong Cork accent. The latter became particularly pronounced during the final warm-up in the pavilion before a match, especially if we were playing one of the more 'aristocratic' English teams such as Harlequins. Just before we emerged sweating on the pitch, Pat would roar: 'Remember, lads, there's only one 'um, and that's fuck 'um!' Pat went on to have a distinguished career as a consultant nephrologist and epidemiologist in Newfoundland, and coached the Canadian national rugby team. To this day, I channel his exhortation ahead of challenging situations, reminding myself that 'There's only one 'um . . .'

My years in London broadened my horizons and my mind. Hitherto, my experience of the practice of obstetrics and gynaecology had been in the atmosphere of 1970s Ireland. Contraception was illegal, tubal ligation was unheard of, and no one discussed abortion. It was also extremely unusual to diagnose fetal abnormality in Ireland during pregnancy: ultrasound was used very selectively and, as abortion was illegal, the question of termination for fetal abnormality never arose.

Irish public policy was largely guided by Catholic moral theology. The 1968 papal encyclical *Humanae vitae* had condemned any form of artificial contraception, and the ultra-conservative and powerful John Charles McQuaid had been Catholic archbishop of Dublin for three decades, up to 1971.

The situation in London was radically different. Contraception was freely available and widely prescribed, and tubal ligations were routinely carried out at Queen Charlotte's and the Chelsea Hospital. And I encountered termination of pregnancy for the first time. The British Abortion Act of 1967 had been in operation for ten years or so, and abortions were performed in the Chelsea on a regular basis. Colleagues assumed that, as I was Irish, I would not want to participate in performing abortions, and so I was not asked. In any event, most terminations were done by more senior colleagues.

Up to now I had not given abortion very much thought – because it simply hadn't been relevant to my working life. When I first went to London, my views were quite conservative – unthinkingly so, in many ways moulded by the environment in Ireland. In London, however, abortion was not a taboo subject, so I had to figure out what I really felt about it.

One of my close friends at the hospital regularly performed terminations, including those arising from fetal abnormalities, such as anencephaly, conditions where the baby has no hope of survival and will die around the time of birth. Over the course of long conversations, he explained how illegal backstreet or self-induced abortions had been the leading cause of maternal mortality in England and Wales prior to 1967. Many illegal abortions had been carried out by injecting poisonous solutions into the uterus or inserting objects intended to dislodge the fetus. Some women had resorted to throwing themselves down stairs or taking herbal compounds or poisons. He told me about the difficult individual circumstances of women seeking terminations, and described how they had come to their decisions. I felt more comfortable looking after women who were having terminations for fetal abnormalities following my discussions with him.

It seemed obvious that one's views are formed by one's environment. The friend with whom I had such enlightening conversations was Jewish and a Londoner. I realized that, had I not been born a Catholic in Ireland, I would almost certainly have had a different view on the ethics of human reproduction. After nearly five years in London and having had to engage in some serious reflection on key aspects of the practice of obstetrics and gynaecology, I was returning to Ireland with a more considered and liberal perspective.

In 1981 I took up a post as registrar in Holles Street and the following year I was appointed to a three-year appointment as one of two assistant masters. We rotated monthly between the obstetric and gynaecological services. Responsibilities included daily rounds of the labour and antenatal wards, organizing the weekly clinical conference, attending antenatal clinics, teaching junior doctors, medical students and student midwives, research, and organizing the duty roster for our more junior colleagues.

There were also two registrars with whom we shared the duty roster. When holidays and study leave were taken into account, we worked a 1:3 rota, and sometimes a 1:2 rota. In other words, we were each on-duty in the hospital for a 24-hour period every two or three days. A weekend on-duty started early Friday morning, and we worked continuously, sleeping when we could snatch some time, for seventy-two hours, until Monday morning. On the Monday morning we would do our regular Monday morning duties and, if lucky, get home sometime on Monday afternoon or evening to sleep. In retrospect, it looks like a savage regime, and hours like this are now completely prohibited.

At the time of the 1983 referendum on the Eighth Amendment I was working day and night in Holles Street, and the campaign passed me by almost completely. Looking back, I find this ironic, given how central a role it played in my later life.

At the NMH in the early 1980s between 7,000 and 8,000 babies were born annually. Since I had first worked there in the mid 1970s the Caesarean section rate had gone up to 6 per cent, between 400 and 500 sections each year.

The epidural rate in first-time mothers had gone from almost zero in the mid 1970s to 8 per cent, and to 2 per cent in those who had already had a baby.

Ultrasound was in the early stages of development and was not performed routinely in all pregnancies. Nevertheless, more than 6,000 scans were done annually (now the figure is in excess of 30,000).

Dermot MacDonald had succeeded Declan Meagher as master of Holles Street in 1977, and under his leadership we were at the forefront of important international research. There was worldwide controversy about the benefit of continuous electronic fetal heart-rate monitoring (EFM) of the baby during labour. Some doctors, especially in the United States, were convinced that monitoring all babies in labour in this way would reduce both the prevalence of cerebral palsy and the number of still-births. Dr MacDonald was interested in this debate and decided to undertake a clinical trial to compare continuous EFM with intermittent auscultation – that is, listening to the baby's heartbeat intermittently with a stethoscope, a practice performed by the midwifery staff.

In association with Oxford University and the UK's National Perinatal Epidemiology Unit, MacDonald was the driver behind the Dublin Fetal Heart-Rate Monitoring Trial, the largest of its kind ever conducted. It was funded by the National Maternity Hospital Research Fund from mid 1981 to mid 1983. The trial involved 12,964 women who were randomized to either continuous EFM or intermittent auscultation. It was made possible by our AML protocols, as every woman in labour had her own personal midwife for the duration of the labour.

My role was to review each of the fetal heart-rate traces in the women who had had continuous EFM, without knowing the outcome of the labour, and to classify them as ominous, suspicious, non-reassuring, reassuring or unclassifiable. Every morning, before doing anything else, I reviewed all traces from the previous twenty-four hours in the hospital. In total I reviewed over 4,000 over the duration of the study. The results of the trial were published in the *American Journal of Obstetrics and Gynecology* in July 1985. We showed that, in a low-risk group of women, continuous EFM did not reduce the incidence of still-birth, neonatal death or cerebral palsy.

Despite our conclusions, continuous EFM is almost universal practice in hospitals around the world now. Fear of litigation is one reason. The failure to change practice in the face of good scientific evidence is an interesting example of how people, doctors included, find it hard to accept something that goes against their in-built biases.

Ireland in the 1980s was a time of recession and political instability, with high unemployment and emigration and declining standards of living. Ireland, indeed, was then regarded as 'the sick man of Europe'. As the economy deteriorated, there was an embargo on public sector employment, which meant that there were no jobs for people like me who had completed their training and were looking for a consultant post. I had been considering working in the United States anyway, and the embargo tipped the balance.

The Dublin Fetal Heart-Rate Monitoring Trial generated huge international interest, and my participation in it was of great assistance in securing a post. Finding myself with three offers – one near Toronto, another in California and a third in Texas – I chose the University of Texas at the Texas Medical Center (TMC) in Houston, because Dr Robert Creasy, an internationally renowned researcher into premature birth, was starting there as chairman at the end of 1984. I was interested to see what changes he would make, and how he would make them.

I arrived in Texas in August 1984 on a special visa that allowed me to work as a visiting professor. My wife Frances and our one-year-old daughter Zoë came a month later. I moved into an apartment with Dr Creasy, as it happened, as he had only recently arrived from San Francisco and was also awaiting the arrival of his family. Creasy was an Episcopalian, and we had many discussions about the influence of upbringing on the formation of our approaches to ethical issues relating to the practice of obstetrics and gynaecology, in particular abortion. These conversations and exposure to another point of view further helped me to develop a more liberal attitude towards abortion.

I was working at the University of Texas's Hermann Hospital, part of TMC. My responsibilities were the management of the labour ward, antenatal and gynaecology clinics, teaching and research, and a small private practice. Although the case of *Roe v. Wade* in 1973 had led to legalization of abortion in the United States, the law in Texas was still restrictive. No early abortions were performed in the hospital, and later abortions, where the mother's life or health was at risk, or in the case of fetal anomalies, were very unusual. In my time in Texas the question of whether or not to terminate a pregnancy never arose.

In Texas I encountered the local equivalent of Irish doctors giving women the pill for, supposedly, irregular menstrual cycles. Some of my TMC colleagues had admitting rights to a hospital owned by a Catholic order. They explained to me that, to circumvent objections by the nuns and the ethics committee, they would describe a tubal ligation performed at the time of a Caesarean section as 'uterine isolation'. They thought this amusing; I thought it hypocritical. But then weren't colleagues doing something similar in Ireland to get around restrictions arising from Catholic teaching?

The TMC was vast, effectively a city in itself with several hospitals across the campus. As well as the Hermann Hospital, there was the Texas Children's Hospital, Baylor University Medical Center and the MD Anderson Cancer Center. It seems strange today, but this was the first time that I had encountered such an open acknowledgement of cancer as a disease. In Ireland the word 'cancer' was rarely used then when dealing with patients or relations. Patients would be admitted for mysterious 'tests'. They might have 'inflammation', or maybe a 'tumour' or a 'lump' would be acknowledged, or they would be told 'things don't look good'. In Texas, cancer was cancer.

The American system could not have been more different from the European public system. Contracts were renewed on an annual basis and appointment to a permanent position could take years to achieve. At the end of each year the chairman would invite me and my colleagues into his office, individually, to discuss our performance. He would tell us how much we had cost in salary, pension contributions, heating, light, insurance and secretarial assistance. On the credit side, he would review our contribution to the department by way of research grants, private practice and fee income. Those of us lucky enough to be in surplus were offered a bonus, whereas those who were costing the department more than they were bringing in were advised that their contract would not be renewed the next year unless matters improved. It certainly provided an incentive to work hard.

When I arrived in Houston, because of the income generated for the department, obstetric ultrasounds were performed by the department of radiology, and not by the department of obstetrics and gynaecology. There ensued a turf war but the ob-gyn department won out in the end, and performing ultrasound scans was one of the ways I was able to generate funds for the department.

The American attitude to holidays was also something of a surprise to me. Several months after arriving my wife and I decided to take our young daughter to Key West for a week. I booked a nice hotel and was looking forward to the trip. The chairman heard about this and came into my office one day and said: 'I hear you are taking a vacation.' I replied with great enthusiasm that we were going to Key West and how excited we all were by the trip. He looked at me in amazement and informed me that that was not the way things worked. He explained to me that normal practice was that no annual leave, or at most one week, was taken in the first year. In the second year, one took two weeks, three weeks in the third year and so on.

I said to him that if that was the case I would go insane, as I felt it necessary to take a break every so often to recharge the batteries. I explained to him that this was the way things worked in Europe, and that I would find it extremely difficult to change. He wasn't particularly happy but accepted my explanation, and we had a wonderful week in Key West. I continued with the European approach to time off, much to the amusement and envy of my colleagues.

Soon after I arrived, I was made director of the labour ward. This gave me a certain degree of authority, although this was difficult to exercise, as there were a lot of different groups that guarded their independence. Hermann Hospital was independent and privately owned, but the University was tasked with running its obstetrics and gynaecological service. In theory this meant that the University's department of obstetrics set the standards and protocols of care, and all doctors, both from the University and those with admitting rights, were supposed to adhere to those standards and protocols. In practice there were a number of fully private obstetricians, and also a group practice of obstetricians, who had admitting rights, and they would manage their patients' labours in their own fashion. So there were several different regimes of care depending on which obstetrician, or group of obstetricians, the woman was attending. I did not find this satisfactory.

Colleagues in Texas were particularly interested in the low Caesarean section rate at the NMH, which at the time was 4.3 per cent compared with an average of 22 per cent in the US. Because I came directly from the NMH there was particular interest in AML, and I set about trying to convince the chairman and faculty members that it was reasonable to attempt to introduce the practice to see if it would result in a reduction in Caesarean section rates.

Immediately I ran into a challenge. One of the main features of AML is the provision of an individual midwife for each woman in labour, but this was not possible in Houston, because midwives in the European sense did not exist in the US, where birth was far more medicalized. Instead, labour ward nurses looked after women in labour, but they were not qualified to conduct deliveries. The resident medical staff conducted all the deliveries, performing the same function as midwives in Ireland. It was not a good system: in the course of labour the nurse might build up a good relationship with the mother, but at the point of delivery a junior doctor, whom the mother had not met before, would arrive and conduct the delivery.

Attending obstetricians, equivalent to consultants in the Irish system, were expected to be present at all deliveries, mainly to observe, but to be ready to step in should problems develop. I soon discovered that this was also for insurance purposes. First, to ensure that the correct insurance company for private patients or Medicaid for uninsured patients would be billed appropriately. Second, if the relevant insurance company learned that a consultant had not attended the delivery, they would refuse to pay the hospital and the doctor.

Still, I gained approval from the ethics committee of the University to conduct a research protocol to see if a form of AML would safely reduce the incidence of Caesarean section in the hospital. An initial analysis was conducted over two six-monthly periods to measure Caesarean section rates, and AML was then introduced. The overall Caesarean section rate declined from 23 and 25 per cent in the two six-month control periods to 20 and 17.7 per cent respectively following the introduction of AML.

There was a lot of anxiety, among the faculty in particular, that the introduction of AML would result in more adverse outcomes for the babies, primarily because of concerns regarding the effect of oxytocin. Reassuringly, however, there were no differences in perinatal outcome for the babies following the introduction of AML.

One of the most important parts of AML was the weekly audit of outcome for all relevant mothers. Involvement of the residents in this audit process was an integral part of the protocol of AML, and it served an important teaching role. (Many hospitals around the world have tried to introduce AML, but they have never been completely successful, because the full package has not been implemented. Most studies have concentrated on using different regimes of oxytocin but have omitted to emphasize the importance of antenatal education, the allocation of a personal midwife to each woman in labour and especially the weekly audit.)

One of my first private patients was a lawyer, married to another lawyer. She needed a forceps delivery. As I was preparing to do this, her husband came to stand behind me and asked if he could videotape the delivery. This caught me by surprise. I realized that he was not trying to capture the happy moment. I had to think on my feet. I concluded that if I made a mess of the delivery and he sued me, I could show the video to my insurance company and advise them that they should settle the case. On the other hand, if the delivery was uncomplicated and they sued me, I could ask them to produce the video in support of my defence. So I agreed. The delivery was uncomplicated and they didn't sue. It was certainly very different to what I had experienced during my training. (Mind you, that highly litigious environment was good preparation for what would transpire in Ireland in years to come.)

An experience with another private patient brought home to me one of the worst problems with the American system of healthcare. She had severe diabetes, which she was finding very difficult to control as an outpatient. I advised her that I needed to admit her urgently to get her blood sugar levels under control; when blood sugars in pregnancy are too high, it can have a serious effect on the baby, and damage to the mother's eyes and kidneys is a very real risk. Her insurance, however, did not cover inpatient admission, so I had no choice but to refer her to the local charity hospital, where I knew that she would be treated by residents without a huge amount of experience.

This was a sad and frustrating illustration of the cruelty of the American system. I had been aware of the gross inequalities in the US healthcare system, but experiencing the reality of it was an unpleasant shock.

The University of Texas Medical School was extremely wealthy. In the distant past the University had been left several million acres of scrubland in western Texas. Oil had been discovered on the land, and the resulting revenues underwrote the massive Permanent University Fund (PUF). In 1981 oil generated $262 million for the University. The fund, which held in excess of a billion dollars at the time I was there, could be used only for capital projects, however, and not for current expenditure. Thus University of Texas buildings were absolutely magnificent, with no expense spared on their construction. I wondered how that money could have been better used for research or treating poor patients.

I ran a clinic in a poor area of Houston, part of a charitable initiative by the University. It was held in a school building, as most of the patients were schoolgirls. They were all black. The school itself was surrounded by wide tracts of bare scrub grass on which stood dilapidated wooden shacks, many of which had no electricity. One day I watched a man walking slowly across this area trailed by a woman, his wife or partner. The scene looked like something from a South African township during the apartheid years rather than America.

Black girls and women in Texas and across the US were (and are) much more likely to die from complications of pregnancy than white women for a combination of reasons, including poorer access to good healthcare. It made no sense to me that the richest state in the richest country in the world could not – or would not – provide healthcare for all of its citizens.

These experiences were among the reasons why I realized that a life in medicine in the US was not for me. I wanted to be able to care for patients without having to be concerned about whether or not they could pay and to work in a more compassionate environment. And I missed the high quality and common-sense approach to obstetrics in Ireland. Apart from the practice of obstetrics, I didn't find the sprawl of Houston or the climate particularly attractive. Frances and I were close to our families and missed the social contact with them and our friends. I began to yearn for Holles Street and Ireland.

4.   Fulfilling my life's ambition

Although I had left Holles Street for London and Houston, my affection for it had never left me. Since committing to a career in obstetrics, I had made it my ambition to one day be appointed master there. My move back to Ireland to take up a post in the hospital brought me one step closer to fulfilling that ambition.

In the spring of 1987 the then master, John Stronge, was attending a conference in the United States and came to visit me in Houston. We discussed my possible return to Holles Street, and how I would best be employed. In particular, we discussed my ambition to develop fetal medicine at the hospital. In Texas I had seen the growing importance of fetal medicine and believed that if I could devote time to developing this area in Holles Street, it would enhance the reputation of the hospital and establish it as a national referral centre for complicated pregnancies.

When Holles Street made a position available, it included my appointment as director of the fetal assessment unit, where high-risk pregnancies were supervised. The job offered a salary of less than 20 per cent of what I was earning in Houston and was not officially approved by the Department of Health. Nonetheless, I jumped at it. I was simply delighted to return to an environment where I knew that, professionally, I would feel much more comfortable. My salary was to be supplemented by teaching, and I was appointed a lecturer in UCD's department of obstetrics and gynaecology.

On New Year's Day 1988 I walked through the doors of Holles Street to take up a post in the hospital where I had worked happily as a junior doctor, the hospital to which I would now commit myself for the rest of my working life. I felt that I had come home.

While happy to be back in Ireland with Frances and our four-year-old Zoë, it soon became clear, however, that I had returned at a difficult time for the hospital. The deep recession of the 1980s had required draconian cost-cutting measures, so that staff were stretched and morale was low. Nonetheless, Dr Stronge gave me the go-ahead to develop my plans and asked me to take over the ultrasound service as it related to fetal assessment.

Improvements in fetal medicine particularly assisted treatment of babies who were affected by rhesus incompatibility, a condition where the mother's blood group is rhesus negative and the baby is rhesus positive. The baby may develop severe anaemia, which can be fatal if untreated. As a result of improvements in ultrasound technology, a new technique of directly transfusing blood into the baby's umbilical cord to overcome the problem had been developed, and I was given the task of introducing this to Ireland. (Rhesus disease is much rarer now because of an injection, Anti-D, given to rhesus negative women during pregnancy.)

Initially I sent patients to London for this treatment, but then went over to King's College Hospital to learn how to do the procedure under the supervision of Professor Kypros Nicolaides, a world-famous pioneer in fetal medicine.

The development of direct intrauterine transfusion under ultrasound guidance was a wonderful medical advance, and over the next several years, when I was the only doctor in Ireland carrying out this procedure, I performed over seventy intrauterine transfusions for rhesus disease. Being responsible for the introduction of the fetal medicine service into Ireland remains one of the proudest achievements of my career.

As there was little private obstetric work at the NMH in the late 1980s, after returning to Dublin I set about trying to gain admitting rights to Mount Carmel, then a private maternity hospital. This would give me the ability to deliver babies and perform gynaecological surgery at Mount Carmel. Almost immediately I encountered a problem in the form of a colleague. Perhaps fearful that I would take patients from his own practice, he tried to block me.

I was surprised to be approached by him one Saturday morning in Holles Street. He smoothly assured me that his objection was not personal; it was merely that he felt it important that a principle be upheld, given that I was not a 'properly appointed' consultant. My reply to him was rather less smooth. His attempts to have my rights rescinded were unsuccessful, although he continued periodically to oppose me over the years – 'on principle' only, of course.

Starting a private practice required me to engage a secretary, and so began one of the most rewarding relationships of my professional life. I was lucky enough to employ Averil Priestman, who remains with me to this day, more than thirty years later. With her warm personality and 'no problem' approach, she was a phenomenal asset, with many patients saying, only half in jest, that it was Averil they went to see – not me – during their pregnancies. I also had a small gynaecological practice, and among the many patients I saw there was a charming, elderly woman who made the journey from deepest Kerry every six months for a check-up. At each visit she brought a fresh wild salmon, which made me very popular on the domestic front (at least twice a year).

In July 1988 one of the most challenging episodes in the history of Holles Street began with the opening of a landmark legal case in the High Court: *Dunne (a minor) v. National Maternity Hospital*. It was the last medical negligence claim in Ireland to be heard before a jury, and it attracted enormous media and public interest. Above all it was deeply distressing for Mr and Mrs Dunne, who had entered the hospital six years earlier expecting to bring home two healthy children. Instead, one of their sons had died and the other was severely brain damaged.

On Saturday, 20 March 1982, Kay Dunne was admitted to Holles Street in early labour. Her first baby, James, had been born healthy at the hospital in January 1980. Mrs Dunne was expecting twins, and the pregnancy had been uncomplicated. Having driven up from Wicklow with her husband, Willie, she arrived at Holles Street at around 10.30 in the morning. At 5.15 that afternoon her first twin, William, was born but he was unexpectedly in poor condition. He was pale, his muscle tone was poor, and he was shocked-looking and slow to breathe. Following resuscitation, he was transferred to the neonatal intensive care unit. Fifteen minutes later the second twin, Martin, was delivered still-born. He showed signs of maceration, a process that occurs after death and indicates that death has taken place some hours or days before birth.

The hospital's assessment, based on the medical evidence, was that Martin had died before Mrs Dunne's arrival, and that the process leading to his death had caused irreversible brain damage in his brother William, who then developed a severe form of cerebral palsy. However, Kay Dunne was convinced that both babies were alive when she entered Holles Street, and that Martin had died during the day. She described an episode of 'tumultuous' fetal movements at around 1.40 p.m. and was certain that she had felt both twins moving.

This was, understandably, deeply distressing to the Dunne parents. They were sure that Martin's death and William's catastrophic brain injury must have been due to a mistake on someone's part, and, against great odds and at considerable financial cost (including selling their house to raise money), they took an action against the hospital and Reginald Jackson, the consultant whom Mrs Dunne had been attending.

From the beginning I was uneasy about the progress of the case. On the morning proceedings opened, I attended a pre-trial consultation at the Four Courts. As the hospital and Dr Jackson were separately insured, there were two defence teams. These teams met in different rooms and did not appear to consult each other. Barristers acting for the hospital asked the usual difficult questions of the doctors at our meeting, but I detected an air of defensiveness, and a rather worrying reluctance to engage fully with the questions.

It was felt that my experience with the Dublin Fetal Heart-Rate monitoring trial, as well as medicolegal cases in America, would be useful for the hospital. I was called as an expert witness to give my opinion on a fetal heart-rate tracing that had run for approximately thirty-five minutes immediately prior to William's birth. I gave evidence that the tracing showed that the fetal heart-rate was normal. In other words, there was no evidence that William was suffering from lack of oxygen during labour.

From the outset the hospital's position was that there had been what is known as a twin transfusion event following Martin's sudden death. This is a spontaneous event where the donor twin – in this case William – loses blood and experiences a catastrophic drop in blood pressure, and the recipient twin – Martin – receives too much blood by transfusion into his circulation. The hospital maintained that as a result of this event by the time Mrs Dunne was admitted Martin had died and William had suffered brain damage as a result of the drop in blood pressure, which had reduced the circulation to his brain. A serious underlying problem with the case was Holles Street's over-confidence in its position, which led to poor preparation. The hospital perhaps hadn't quite appreciated how, particularly in a case with a lot of technical evidence, doubts could be cast on its interpretation of events. And they possibly hadn't allowed for the natural sympathy a jury of twelve ordinary citizens would have for parents who had experienced such a traumatic situation. Instead of being complacent they needed to work hard to explain themselves respectfully. But that was not quite how the hospital approached it. Barristers for the defence were embarrassed on several occasions by contradictory evidence given by representatives of the hospital.

The hospital maintained that the policy at the time was to listen to only one fetal heart during labour in the case of a twin pregnancy, as it was thought impossible to distinguish between fetal hearts in a twin pregnancy. If Martin had already died before admission to the hospital, it wouldn't have mattered that only one fetal heartbeat was listened for. This was met with incredulity by British experts appearing for the Dunnes, and when a UK expert was brought on by the defence to argue that such a policy was reasonable, under cross-examination it transpired that the policy in his own hospital was to listen for two fetal hearts. (During the subsequent retrial of the case it emerged that the policy of listening to only one heart during the course of a labour with twins was not in fact adhered to by the midwives at Holles Street. With the help of their solicitor the Dunnes managed to track down ten women who could describe how, when giving birth to twins in Holles Street, in the year before and after Mrs Dunne, the heartbeats of both twins had been monitored during their labours.)

The discovery process, whereby documents are sought from the hospital, was incomplete, and, as more information emerged as the case went on, the hospital's defence was further undermined. The hospital also inadvertently denied the existence of the student midwife who had actually delivered William. Possibly due to volume of work at the hospital, they had simply forgotten about the young nurse – but, given her role in the birth of Mrs Dunne's twins, and the importance of the case, it was careless in the extreme not to have accounted for every person involved. All in all, it was a shambles of the hospital's own making.

The case for the Dunnes, on the other hand, came across as coherent and consistent, and clearly it was an account of events that made sense to the jury, because at the end of the three-week trial it found in favour of the family and they were awarded more than a million Irish pounds.

The hospital appealed the case to the Supreme Court, and a retrial was ordered on the basis of a legal technicality. Recognizing the hopelessness of defending the case, after sixteen days the hospital settled, with the complete exoneration of Dr Jackson. The original award was reduced to IR£400,000. All costs were awarded against Holles Street, including the Dunnes' legal bills of more than IR£200,000. William was made a ward of court, with the money to be invested by the court and drawn down by his parents as William needed it.

In the wake of the case and its damaging consequences for Holles Street's reputation, the Workers' Party Deputy Pat Rabitte observed in a Dáil debate in May 1990 that 'the bizarre progress of the case raises profound issues of credibility about the administration of our National Maternity Hospital.' Given the recession and declining birth numbers, there was talk of closing one of the three Dublin maternity hospitals, and for a time it looked like Holles Street's days were numbered.* Various people called for a public inquiry. The then Minister for Health, Dr Rory O'Hanlon, said that it was a matter for the hospital to initiate such an inquiry, since he had no jurisdiction over what was a voluntary organization. The executive committee of the hospital commissioned a report from Dr Geoffrey Chamberlain, professor of obstetrics and gynaecology at St George's Hospital Medical School at the University of London.

Professor Chamberlain delivered his report in the autumn of 1990. His overall finding was that the severe underfunding of the hospital was the source of many of the recent problems, which, he observed, did not 'stem [from] lack of professional regard but overstretching of facilities'. He then went on to highlight a number of specific issues. I had worked with Professor Chamberlain during my time training in London and as, by now, I knew I would be taking up the mastership the following January, I travelled over to meet him and was able to tease out his recommendations in detail.

He advised a more liberal approach to the use of epidurals for pain relief (a policy I was already fully intending to implement as soon as I became master a few months later) and suggested that there should

---

* In 1992 Minister for Health John O'Connell, a successor of Rory O'Hanlon in the portfolio, confirmed to me that serious consideration had been given to closing Holles Street in the previous couple of years.

be a closer coordination of midwives' notes, something that was immediately adopted in Holles Street. Previously midwives' records had not been included in the main hospital notes, something that had been a source of irritation to me over the years when I had to go looking for their separate notes. I also felt that this approach diminished the role of the midwife.

In recommending more extensive use of ultrasound for the diagnosis of fetal abnormality, Chamberlain noted that he was 'sensitive to the differences in philosophy about termination of pregnancy between our two countries', but accurately predicted that, as more women learned about the possibility of diagnosing abnormality, demand for terminations would increase.

Some of his recommendations were more reflective of the British approach to obstetrics, with Holles Street midwives, for example, judged as having too much authority on the labour ward. The suggestion, therefore, was that there should be greater involvement of junior doctors. I did not agree with this. An experienced midwife is a much better judge of the progress of a labour, and the appropriate point to intervene, than a junior doctor in training.

I have always believed that midwives and doctors should work together as a team and have never subscribed to the concepts of exclusively 'obstetrician-led' or 'midwifery-led' care. Some women have more complicated pregnancies and labours than others and need more input from doctors. Others don't. No woman should go through a pregnancy without contact with both a midwife and a doctor. One of the features of obstetrics is that complications can arise with little or no warning, particularly during labour. If this happens, it is much better that the doctor called is not a stranger to the woman. For this reason, it is important that doctors undertake regular ward rounds of the delivery ward.

The Dunne case had far-reaching repercussions, not only for the Dunnes themselves, but also in the establishment of what are known as the Dunne Principles. These principles were set out by Chief Justice Thomas Finlay in the Supreme Court judgment and are the legal guidelines on which all cases of medical negligence are still decided in Ireland today.

While it was right that Mr and Mrs Dunne were able to give William the care he needed, they should never have had to go through the trauma of seven years of legal action, with all its associated expense and stress. The state should have a system in place to provide for parents and children in similar circumstances.

I first advocated publicly for reform in this area in an interview with the *Irish Medical Times* in August 1990 when I called for no-fault insurance and said that all parents of a child with a disability should be entitled to support from the state. A few months later, in an interview in the *Sunday Business Post*, I addressed the issue of growing litigation costs, expressing my concern that Ireland was heading in the same direction as the US, where I had seen for myself the high incidence of medical litigation.

It is a human reaction to want to find a reason for a tragic event. This, combined with the lack of state support for families who have children with special needs, and our litigious environment, has led to a situation where, in the years since the Dunne case, the level of negligence claims in obstetric cases has skyrocketed. By 2016, 65 per cent of the €1.6 billion ongoing contingency for claims against the state was for obstetric cases, in particular cerebral palsy. Yet there has been no reduction in rates of cerebral palsy, and nothing on the horizon suggests any development in this regard.

The current system is totally unsatisfactory. In looking for support for their children parents are at the mercy of the legal system. It takes many years for cases to come to court, and we are all too familiar with seeing families outside the High Court expressing relief at having finally settled their case after years of uncertainty. We are struck, of course, by their bravery, tenacity and determination to do their best for their children, but in my view it would be a far better system for the state to provide a high standard of care to all children with a disability, regardless of the cause.

The Dunne case and the Chamberlain Report made it clear that change and modernization were needed at Holles Street. In the 1980s there had been significant advances in obstetric practice worldwide, particularly in the areas of fetal medicine, ultrasound, minimally invasive gynaecology surgery and neonatal intensive care. I could see the potential for developing these services in Holles Street to modernize the treatments available to women and infants.

The new mastership term would start in January 1991. This was an opportunity for a fresh start and I very much wanted to be in a position to lead the hospital into a new era. So, in May 1990, I stood for election to the mastership. As a result of my time in Houston, in particular, I felt I could bring international experience and financial competence to the role. Above all, I was determined that the environment in Holles Street should be more woman-friendly, modern and in tune with what women themselves wanted.

I could not, of course, be sure of succeeding in my application to become master, and so I also applied for other jobs in the city as they came up. After all, my position at the time was temporary, so I needed a permanent job. After a couple of failures, I was appointed to a post between the Rotunda and Beaumont hospitals, just a couple of weeks before the mastership election in May 1990, and this gave me some security going into the interviews.

There were three candidates for the master's position: Michael Foley, Michael Turner and myself. We were each invited to have dinner individually with the honorary officers of the hospital board – the deputy chairman,* Alex Spain, the incoming honorary secretary, John Meagher, and the honorary treasurer, Brian Davy. Alex Spain was a well-known and successful businessman who had been managing partner of the accountants Stokes, Kennedy, Crowley. His father, also Alex, was an obstetrician who had been master of Holles Street in the 1940s. John Meagher was on the board of Independent Newspapers and ran Irish Marketing Surveys, while Brian Davy was one of the principals of Davy Stockbrokers. Brian's father, James, had been on the Holles Street board for almost fifty years, holding the position of honorary secretary for forty-two years before being appointed deputy chairman for five years. The dinner was held in a private dining room in Alex Spain's office on Mount Street, and its purpose was to explore each of our ambitions for the future of the hospital. While it wasn't to see how we held our knives and forks, it was, effectively, trial by dinner.

In the wake of the Dunne case, we were all acutely aware that it would be essential to restore the hospital's reputation during the next

---

*Effectively the deputy chair of the board (or executive committee) acts as its chair, because, by custom, the official chair, the Catholic archbishop of Dublin, does not participate in board meetings.

mastership term. The public perception of the hospital at that time was of an austere, conservative and distant institution. I argued the need for a policy of modernization and openness.

A week later, we were each interviewed formally. The job of the interview committee was to recommend a candidate to the 100 governors of the hospital, who would then vote to confirm if they were in agreement with that recommendation. Immediately after the vote in the hospital's boardroom, the decision was announced to the candidates and staff.

It took until after I retired in 2016 before I discovered what had happened after the interviews. Brian Davy had chaired the interview committee, and at the end of the first round of discussions it was a dead heat between myself and one other. Brian would have to exercise the casting vote. He was reluctant to do this, decided to have a second round of discussions, and was relieved when one member changed his mind in favour of me. His heart sank, however, when another member then changed his mind in favour of the other candidate. So Brian had to exercise the casting vote after all, and I was fortunate to get the recommendation.

I was elated to be appointed. I knew where I would be and what I would be doing for the next seven years. I could implement the plans I had been formulating over the previous decade.

The mastership model of hospital management dates from 1745, when Bartholomew Moss founded the Rotunda Hospital. Over the years the model has evolved to its present-day arrangement whereby the master of each of the three Dublin maternity hospitals – the Rotunda, the Coombe and Holles Street – is elected by the governors for a seven-year term. The master can serve only one term. The first master of the hospital, Sir Andrew Horne, had been in office for thirty years,★ and it was partly to stop this from happening again that the seven-year rule was introduced at Holles Street. The Rotunda and Coombe already had this restriction in place.

★ For the avoidance of doubt, this is contrary to the information included on Holles Street's Wikipedia page, which is incorrect. In the beginning there were two masters. Horne was joint master from 1894 to 1924 and three separate masters were in office with him in those years.

The master has corporate responsibility for everything that happens in the hospital, including standards of patient care, finances and administration. The financial and administrative aspects are effectively under the guidance of the secretary/manager, assisted by finance and administration staff, but the secretary/manager reports to the master. Similarly, the matron of the hospital (now known as director of nursing and midwifery) also reports to the master. In turn, the master reports to the executive committee of the board of governors, which meets every month.

The position of the master carries considerable authority within the hospital, and this allows each master to decide on the priorities for their term of office. What makes it so effective and differentiates it from the CEO role in other hospitals is that the master is always a practising doctor who understands intimately the business of medicine. One of the benefits of a seven-year term is that it provides enough time to make a mark, but if problems occur it is not so long that the hospital cannot recover from a poor incumbent. The master is, effectively, the captain of the team, or master of the ship.

Following my election, and before starting the job in January 1991, I attended meetings of the executive committee as an observer. I had made it clear that one of my first priorities would be to regain the trust of the public after the Dunne case and restore the reputation of the hospital. Holles Street had been buffeted by a combination of events in the preceding few years. The country was emerging from a deep recession that resulted in severe financial constraints on any developments in the hospital and an embargo on the appointment of staff. There was genuine concern about the future of the hospital, and it was thought that women were being put off attending Holles Street as a consequence of the Dunne case, because of the restriction on epidural pain relief in labour (discussed below) and because of a general impression of Catholic conservatism.

My new role would inevitably involve engagement with the media, so the executive decided that I should undergo media training. My first trial television interview at Carr Communications did not go well. In response to aggressive questioning I was defensive. I was advised not to score points off the interviewer or rise to references to the past. Answers should be pitched to the proverbial intelligent fourteen-year-old. Other good advice was not to attempt to defend the indefensible, and always to stick to the message I wanted to convey, irrespective of the line of questioning.

Further tips related to my appearance and I was advised always to shave before going on television, to sit straight on to the interviewer, to wear a pastel-coloured shirt (without stripes) and a pale grey suit, and never to wear a stripy tie. I wasn't so sure about the pale suit, but a second trial interview went better and I was considered 'trained'.

From the outset my approach to media inquiries was always to respond to a phone call (or later a text). I commented on the record – or didn't, if I had nothing to say or it was not appropriate for me to comment. Sometimes I provided background information. Early in my mastership the *Irish Medical Times* suggested that 'medics who constantly moan about being misrepresented should take a leaf from [my] book and have the self-confidence to treat the media as something other than a particularly nasty virus that has to be contained.' This rather colourful line had more than a nugget of truth. I have never regarded the media as 'the enemy', but rather as an essential pillar of a functioning democracy. (That's not to say that journalists don't make mistakes.)

From the beginning of my mastership, I implemented a planned communications strategy intended to demonstrate greater openness and engagement with the public and the media. I gave many interviews in which I emphasized that the hospital was beginning a new, liberal approach on several fronts. I reiterated that 'the most important person in the hospital is the woman walking through the door. It was built for the women: it wasn't built for me or for anybody else.' It was their hospital, not mine.

I started by announcing that epidural analgesia would now be available on request to any woman who wanted it. An epidural is a superb form of pain relief, nothing less and nothing more. John Stronge had been of a conservative bent when it came to the provision of epidurals in labour, because of concerns that it would increase the rate of intervention during labour; in 1988 only 15 per cent of women having their first baby received an epidural for pain relief. Of the 306 women who had a Caesarean section that year, only 11 per cent had their Caesareans performed under epidural analgesia, as opposed to general anaesthesia.

Having just two consultant anaesthetists on the staff, because of cutbacks, didn't help matters. By 1990 Dr Stronge had succeeded in doubling the number of anaesthetists, but, while the proportion of women undergoing Caesarean section under epidural had increased to 28 per cent in women having their first baby, there had been no change in the rate of epidural for pain relief during labour. By international standards these rates were extremely low, and were a cause of tension between the anaesthetic consultants and Dr Stronge, to say nothing of the frustration felt by women. My experience in London and Houston, however, had taught me that epidurals were not as risky as some more medically conservative doctors believed.

It was one of my key aims as master to liberalize the use of epidural both for pain relief in labour and for Caesarean section, and so I moved immediately to implement the new policy. In the first year of my mastership, the epidural rate rose overall from just under 10 per cent to just over 18 per cent, and it had increased to 30 per cent by 1992. By 1993, 50 per cent of first-time mothers were availing of epidurals.

For some women, going through labour and delivering their baby without any pain relief is an enormously satisfying and fulfilling achievement. But I have never believed that pain is an ennobling experience, and for many other women it can cause long-lasting emotional trauma. I have always felt that women should have a choice about what, if any, form of pain relief they wish for, and also that they should be able to change their mind when faced with the reality of labour. On several occasions I was saddened to come across couples where the man was insisting his partner go through labour without pain relief because that was what 'we decided in *our* birth plan'. I had to suppress the urge to say, 'Sorry, mate, you're not the one in pain – she can have an epidural.' Interference of that kind could indicate a controlling man, and one had to be mindful of the possible consequences of intervening in what might be an emotionally or physically abusive relationship during the fraught circumstances of a difficult labour.

There was a concern that increasing the epidural rate would lead to an increase in Caesarean births or the use of forceps, but this did not happen. During my period as master, Holles Street had one of the highest percentages of natural births – that is, birth without intervention – in Europe. These figures were a tribute to the skills of the midwives in the labour ward. And the relaxation of our policy about giving epidurals gained much media attention, thereby reassuring women about the hospital.

I was determined to keep going, to implement measures that I believed were necessary to help our patients. But I knew that my next task would be more difficult: I wanted to liberalize the hospital's approach to sterilization. So I was on an inevitable collision course with the Catholic Church.

5. Steering the ship at Holles Street

Sterilization was a thorny and controversial subject at Holles Street for years. In 1978 John Stronge's predecessor, Dermot MacDonald, wanted to perform a sterilization operation on a woman who had serious medical and social problems. He informed consultants and other staff, and also the archbishop of Dublin, Dermot Ryan, chairman of the hospital board, of his intention. The archbishop, although he could not agree with MacDonald's plans, did nothing to obstruct him. However, the matron, Una Murphy, wrote a letter of protest to all the governors, including the archbishop, expressing her opposition, and that of a number of her nursing and midwifery staff. Having contacted several other governors, Archbishop Ryan put it to Dr MacDonald that this might be a resigning matter. MacDonald, however, was determined and proceeded with the sterilization, assisted by Declan Meagher, his immediate predecessor, and a number of younger nurses.

The issue was discussed at the next meeting of the executive committee. Professor Eamon de Valera, son of the former President and a devout Catholic, strongly disapproved of the master's action. The meeting was chaired, however, by the deputy chairman, James Davy, then in his eighties, who was very supportive of the master. It appeared that MacDonald had been successful in putting the matter behind him. Yet, at the next meeting of the executive, he came under further attack. He announced that if he was obliged to resign, he would have to give a full account of the reasons at a press conference.

A compromise was reached with the proposal that an ethics committee be formed in order to oversee such matters in the future. The strength of feeling among some in the hospital is illustrated by an incident that occurred a little while later. MacDonald was mowing the grass at home when he accidentally cut off the tops of two fingers on his right hand. He subsequently got a letter from one of his more conservative colleagues, quoting Matthew's Gospel: 'If thy right hand offend thee, cut it off.'

In order to bring clarity to the question of sterilization John Stronge, in conjunction with the ethics committee, laid down a policy expressly forbidding the procedure as a method of family planning. It was permitted only for medical reasons, where it was clear that future pregnancies would be dangerous for a woman.

At the time, the Adelaide, which had a Church of Ireland ethos, was the only hospital in Dublin where sterilizations were performed with no restrictions. There was a two-year waiting list and around 400 were performed annually. Sterilizations in the Rotunda had to be vetted first by their ethics committee, while in the Coombe they were carried out for medical reasons only, although they were also planning at this stage to review their policy. Meanwhile the Mater and St Vincent's strictly enforced a ban on all sterilizations.

In my view, not providing this service was causing considerable hardship for many women. In January 1992 I did an interview with Ursula Halligan for the *Sunday Tribune* and told her that there was now a more liberal attitude among patients, nursing staff and doctors on the issue: 'In general,' I said, 'virtually everyone would be happier if tubal ligation could be offered as a means of family planning.' I also said that I thought it was time for the ethics committee to meet again to consider the issue, and that, since I had become master just over a year previously, more tubal ligations (ten in total) had been carried out than in any previous twelve-month period. 'Every request for tubal ligation has to be seen by me and I interpret the guidelines as sympathetically as possible,' I explained. The article was headlined: 'Maternity Hospital Set to Oppose Church Doctrine'.

My observation of Catholic involvement in Irish hospitals was that religious ideology was rarely a problem in orthopaedics or cardiology, for example, but frequently created serious problems for women's healthcare. A medical source in the Mater told Ursula Halligan that 'Hypothetically, if a woman with a severe heart condition of a life-threatening nature requested a tubal ligation there, she would be refused.' Halligan noted that a woman with such a condition could be treated only in the Mater because the National Cardiac Unit was located there. So in this notional example even cardiology care was indirectly affected. It seemed that when it came to healthcare, women's reproductive capacity was a fixation of the Catholic Church, to the exclusion of their overall well-being.

A couple of weeks after the *Sunday Tribune* interview I talked to Padraig O'Morain at the *Irish Times*. I told him that I had noticed an increase in requests for sterilizations during my time as master, and that I would like the ethics committee to review the guidelines. I also said that I didn't want to put anybody under pressure to act in a way that was contrary to their beliefs. 'We are a non-denominational hospital,'* I said. 'We serve all members of the community and in the light of that and in the light of everybody's beliefs we have to review the situation. But it has to be done in a calm, balanced way and that's what I am trying to achieve.'

In that same interview I also raised the issue of amniocentesis, a test for genetic abnormalities that was not available in the Republic at that time. I suggested that it should be part of the antenatal diagnostic service. 'A lot of women who have had a baby with a problem in the past . . . need to get information on what the risks are for the future. That would be a benefit.' Inevitably, this raised the spectre of the Eighth Amendment and the prohibition on abortion in any circumstances other than those in which the life of the mother was in danger.

Over the course of several months the issue of tubal ligation was debated at the ethics committee – comprising one priest, three doctors, three nurses and two hospital governors – and I reported on progress, or the lack thereof, to the executive each month. I began to tire, however, of the interminable debate, and one evening decided to take the matter into my own hands by unilaterally calling for a vote at an executive committee meeting on whether or not tubal ligation could be provided in the hospital. I had looked around the table at those who were present and calculated that if I called a vote it would be successful. I was correct, and the executive committee agreed that tubal ligation would now be provided, albeit with severe restrictions.

---

* The Catholic archbishop's role as ex-officio chair of the board dates from the hospital's original charter of 1903; the position was established as a reflection of the faith to which the majority of Dubliners then subscribed. Two members of the Dublin City Council were also board members, to represent Dublin's civic society. It is not a Catholic hospital, as the Church does not own it. Although no archbishop has ever exercised his right to chair the executive committee, there is nothing to stop any future archbishop from doing so.

I would have to review every case and countersign each request made by the consultants in the gynaecology clinics, and report on the numbers to the executive committee every month.

I had not given advance warning of the vote to the deputy chairman of the board, Alex Spain. A great supporter of mine, he understood the respective roles of master and deputy chairman and never interfered with the running of the hospital, but it would be fair to say that I had interfered in his running of the board meeting on that occasion.

Immediately after the meeting, Alex took me aside and told me never to call a vote again without giving him warning. He also pointed out that, whatever one might think about the Catholic Church, it was an organization that had been around for 2,000 years, had survived many scandals and had a global reach. I should be very wary, he warned me, of taking it on. Those were words that I would remember many times in the years ahead.

I knew that this change in policy would bring me into conflict with the Catholic archbishop, Desmond Connell. A few weeks after the executive vote there was a letter to my office requesting that I and the matron attend a meeting with the archbishop in his palace in Drumcondra. It wasn't so much an invitation as a command.

Frankly I was irritated at being summoned by the archbishop. I anticipated that he was going to tell us that we had to stop doing sterilizations, and I felt it was not his place to interfere in the clinical care of patients attending the hospital. Maeve Dwyer, the hospital's newly appointed matron, and I drove to Drumcondra together for our audience with Archbishop Connell. Maeve was an extraordinarily supportive colleague who was totally on board with providing sterilizations at Holles Street. For the occasion I had chosen to wear a suit lined in a rather fetching shade of ecclesiastical purple. Not that this sartorial flourish would cut any ice, as it turned out.

Arriving at the archbishop's palace, a young priest showed us into a gloomy ante-room, asked us to wait and disappeared through a heavy wooden door. We sat in silence for ten minutes before he reappeared and led us into a large meeting room dominated by a large highly polished table. Archbishop Connell and Auxiliary Bishop James Moriarty sat together on one side of the table. They did not get up to greet us. Maeve and I sat on the other. There was no chit-chat about traffic or the weather or any attempt at small talk to break the ice. The atmosphere was not friendly. I had a strong impression that we were being viewed almost as a different species.

Bishop Moriarty did most of the talking and got straight to the point in relation to the introduction of sterilization in Holles Street. What I was doing, in their view, was resulting in women having operations that were not medically indicated and were therefore unjustified. Their argument was based on the orthodox Catholic doctrine that the marital act, sexual intercourse, had to remain 'open to the gift of new life'.

I put the position that psychological or social reasons were both important and acceptable grounds for tubal ligation. They rejected that. I stressed that, in my opinion, the operations were justified, and that the women attending the hospital chose to undergo the procedures for very good reasons and did not regard them as an assault, as they had implied. I also informed them that I was not going to reverse the decision, as I felt that that would not be in the best interests of women. Sterilization, I said, was a matter between a woman and her doctor, and the Catholic Church should not interfere in the doctor–patient relationship. I made it clear that, while I respected their opinion, I was the doctor with responsibility for caring for the women attending the National Maternity Hospital, and they were not.

There was an ocean of mutual incomprehension between us across the table. After about half an hour of discussion it was clear that there was going to be no meeting of minds, and Bishop Moriarty brought the meeting to an end. The atmosphere had been chilly to begin with; by the end it was arctic. They continued to sit as we left the room. We drove away, relieved that the meeting was behind us and with a sense of returning to the real world. After leaving Drumcondra that day, I never heard from the archbishop on this or any other subject again.

There was no opposition from the staff and I had the support of enough members of the executive to save me from being forced to consider resignation, as had been Dermot MacDonald's experience fourteen years earlier. Within the next couple of years I was able to relax the hospital's strict criteria for sterilization and the practice became a normal part of gynaecological care. By 1994 we performed 321 tubal ligations in Holles Street. In my last year as master, 1997, that number was 445. This was a radical change in practice, but the numbers showed that it had addressed an unmet need.

Of course, while radical policy changes such as the provision of sterilization were eye-catching, both internally and to the public, my life as master was mainly about the day-to-day rhythm of the hospital and being as present and aware as I could be of everything that was going on in it.

My working day was long and intense. I developed a routine that saw me arrive in the hospital well before 8 a.m. and go straight to the labour ward to check on the night's activities. I then took back to my office a record of the labours of all the women who had delivered in the previous twenty-four hours and reviewed each case individually. A key element of review was an analysis of the partogram of every woman who had delivered. Partograms had been developed by O'Driscoll during his mastership as part of his focus on improving labour outcomes. A partogram is a way of recording important data during labour. These details are entered against time on a sheet of paper. Measurements such as cervical dilation, fetal heart-rate, duration of labour, and the outcome of labour for both the mother and baby can be included. Essentially it tells the story of every labour. Using a ruler and a coloured pencil, I drew lines on each of the partograms, outlining the rate of cervical dilation and whether or not oxytocin or an epidural had been administered.

I liked to show visitors what I was doing and they were amazed that I had not delegated this apparently banal activity to a junior doctor. I used to delight in pointing out to them that the *raison d'être* of the hospital was the care of women giving birth, and that as master it was my job to know in precise detail what happened to every woman who passed through its doors. I considered it vitally important that the master's main focus was on the women in the hospital and not on other non-clinical matters. Knowing how much time American maternity hospital chiefs spent focusing on anything but the women giving birth, I particularly liked making this point to visitors from the US.

My partogram reviews were sent back to the labour ward, and midwives and junior staff would check them to see if I had commented on the management of any of their cases. They could also review the outcome of labours they had been involved in up to the point of going off-duty. The partograms provided a valuable educational source for midwives, medical students and doctors. They also alerted all staff that everything that had happened in the night would be reviewed by the master early the next morning. I worked on the basis that people tend to take more pride in their jobs and do them better when the boss takes an active and constructive interest in what they are doing.

Following my review of the labour ward activity, my next call was the operating theatre, to review overnight activity there. There would usually have been emergency Caesarean sections or ectopic pregnancy surgery, and I would want to know exactly what had happened.

Twice a week, I did a ward round of the antenatal inpatients. These were women who had been admitted for a variety of reasons including complicated twin or triplet pregnancies, high blood pressure, hyperemesis (vomiting excessively in pregnancy and requiring hydration and other treatment), heart disease, diabetes or other conditions, or those who were having an induction of labour. The round was a review of the patients in order to make decisions, but it was also useful for teaching and to immerse myself in the daily activities of the hospital.

One rather timid woman who had several admissions to hospital during her pregnancy sticks in my mind. The junior doctors were at a loss to explain the reasons for her repeated admissions, all associated with vague symptoms. I suspected domestic abuse, and one day, with the curtains drawn around her, I asked quietly, 'How are things at home?' She started to cry and it became clear that her repeated admissions were in fact a cry for help. She was immediately referred to the hospital social workers. Ward rounds like this were important for keeping in touch with the realities of life for the women attending the hospital.

I also did a twice-weekly ward round of the postnatal patients. This was in the nature of a 'meet and greet' and gave me a valuable opportunity to see or hear at first hand if the mothers were having any problems. The hospital infrastructure, like that of so many hospitals in Ireland, was inadequate for the numbers attending, and I often had cause to apologize for the facilities during my rounds. On one occasion, apologizing to a woman after a particularly busy period, I commented that the ward was 'like Beirut'. (Beirut at the time had been devastated by a lengthy civil war.)

'No, it's not,' she responded. 'I'm from Beirut.' And I realized, not for the first or last time, that from our comparatively privileged position in Ireland, we are apt to exaggerate about our conditions sometimes.

As master, I also conducted a weekly gynaecology clinic that also involved meeting parents who had had an unfortunate outcome or who had complaints about their care. It is recognized that people who live through distressing, traumatic experiences do not always form a clear memory of events. I remember one woman who had lost her baby by miscarriage at eighteen weeks. She was on the antenatal ward and was extremely upset because she believed she had delivered her baby, alone, into the toilet. This had not happened: in fact she had been transferred to the delivery ward and delivered the baby in a single room with a midwife present. She was, however, certain of what she remembered, and was distressed. She made a formal complaint, and I met with her and her husband some weeks later to discuss it. I had checked the exact sequence of events with the midwifery staff beforehand.

I listened sympathetically to her description of what had happened and then explained to her what had actually occurred. Her husband corroborated my account. But this clarity caused her even more upset and had the opposite effect to what I had intended. I wondered afterwards whether I had helped her at all, or whether I had inadvertently increased her grief. She had a narrative in her mind and I had destroyed it. Years later I was reassured by a psychologist friend that the woman, with the passage of time, would probably come to realize that the delivery of her baby was more dignified than she had originally thought and that would be a source of comfort to her. I hope that that was the case.

On another occasion I came across a woman in tears in the sister's office. I asked what was wrong and she explained that her gynaecological operation had been cancelled because the surgeon was sick and there was no one else to do it for her. I said I would do the operation for her the next morning. The operation went well, but later that night she began to bleed internally, a rare complication. I had to return her to the operating theatre at 1 a.m. and with the help of a colleague we managed to stop the bleeding. Eventually, I left Holles Street at 3 a.m. and, driving close to home, nearly ran over a black cat that ran across the road in front of me. Not a good sign, I thought, before shortly afterwards coming across three youths walking behind a teenage girl. It looked suspicious and I was concerned for her safety, so I pulled over and rolled down the window to see if she was okay or wanted a lift. She took one look at me, told me I was a dirty old man and to 'fuck off'. The three lads laughed, so I drove on somewhat chastened, and reflecting that no good deed goes unpunished.

In my first six months as master, I thought that the relentless workload was going to kill me. Slowly, however, I learned the benefits of delegation and got better at managing my time. I was helped in my task by Bernardine O'Driscoll, whose institutional knowledge was unsurpassed. As secretary down the years to six masters, including Shane Higgins today (I was her second), she was (and is) an absolute rock, totally reliable and discreet, and loved by all. She has a great sense of humour and always made the master's office a relaxed place, no matter what was going on outside. Nothing ever fazed Bernardine, who was wonderfully phlegmatic. From time to time she would answer the phone to an agitated member of the public. To my intense amusement she would murmur soothingly as she listened, putting the phone down every now and again to continue her work. At intervals she would pick it up again and continue to placate her caller, rolling her eyes at me as she did so. She was also, however, extremely competent at dealing with sensitive issues, a regular occurrence in the master's office.

Early in my term I came up with a plan to improve conditions at the hospital and raise some revenue at the same time. I decided to convert some rooms in what was part of the nurses' home into private rooms for postnatal patients with insurance. The rooms on the first floor of the hospital facing Merrion Square were largely empty, as most nurses now lived outside the hospital. Having some modern private rooms would have the dual function of improving the image of the hospital while also providing a significant revenue stream, which, among other things, could be used to refurbish other parts of the hospital. The Department of Health controlled the number of private rooms allowable in publicly funded hospitals, but since I wasn't increasing the total complement – just replacing some scruffy old ones scattered around the hospital – I didn't have to get departmental approval. Development of what became known as the Merrion Wing also allowed us to meet a recommendation of the Chamberlain Report, as it gave us space to reconfigure the very large wards into smaller four- and six-bed units.

Una Murphy, the matron at the time, had been unimpressed with my plans. 'Every master says he is going to do that,' she said dismissively. We did not see eye to eye, and nor was this my first run-in with her. Earlier in my career, when I was an assistant master, she had stopped me in the corridor one day and told me, somewhat brusquely, to get my hair cut. I had been working incredibly long hours for a few weeks and my hair was indeed a bit long. I had intended getting it cut the very next day, but, of course, now felt obliged to put it off for another few days because of her intervention. Una retired about a year into my mastership, having given thirty-four years of tremendous and loyal service to the hospital. Her successor, Maeve Dwyer, was a fabulous addition to Holles Street, and we got on extremely well together.

With the support of the executive committee and the governors, the IR£500,000 required for the Merrion Wing was lent by individual governors, some of the hospital consultants and a bank. Plans were drawn up for twelve en suite rooms with a separate nursery, and building and fund-raising commenced. The Merrion Wing opened to great fanfare in mid 1992. Within a couple of years the loans were paid off, and the whole endeavour had not cost the state a penny. There was a steady increase in income from private beds over the seven years of my mastership, and hospital income from bed days funded by the insurance companies more than doubled, from just over IR£1 million in 1991 to IR£2.3 million by 1997.

I had hoped, however, that the extra revenue generated by the private rooms could be used to improve the public side of the hospital, but, as the private income of the hospital went up, the allocation from the state went down. This was infuriating and a classic example of a small-minded approach to anyone taking an entrepreneurial spirit in the Irish health service. It was not the last time I felt the 'dead hand' of the Department of Health.

Since the Merrion Wing had been such a success, I planned to do the same for the gynaecology patients and got verbal approval from the secretary of the Department of Health. Yet when it came to proceeding with the project, we were not given the go-ahead. I was subsequently told that the other two maternity hospitals in the city had lobbied against the scheme. Women were the losers.

My ambitions for ongoing development at Holles Street required finance beyond that provided by the state, and so fund-raising became a key objective. There had been little activity in the previous decade, largely because of the deep recession, but, as the economy improved in the 1990s, things changed. Apart from the development of the Merrion Wing, key objectives included the opening of a new neonatal unit and a new fetal assessment unit.

Our first major fund-raising event was a Bloomsday Ball at the RDS in June 1991, an appropriate date, since an episode of James Joyce's *Ulysses*, 'The Oxen of the Sun', is set during a visit by Leopold Bloom to the old Holles Street hospital. The event was a great success and raised a significant amount of money, which was put towards the purchase of equipment for the neonatal unit. The following year it was a fashion show at Jurys Hotel (to raise funds for two ultrasound machines). And the year after that our big event was the premiere of Sir Richard Attenborough's film *Chaplin* at the Savoy Cinema, followed by a party for 800 people in the Gresham Hotel (in aid of the neonatal unit). Attenborough himself was there, as was Taoiseach Albert Reynolds, and various politicians and media folk.

Coming into 1994, our centenary year, I was conscious of the opportunity to alter the hospital's conservative image and to boost staff morale. Alison Stanley joined Director Peggy Maguire in the fund-raising office, and considerable planning went into a huge range of events for the year. The programme had three dimensions – scientific, artistic and social – and our aim was to celebrate the hospital's history and to encourage the widest possible public engagement. Maeve Dwyer was instrumental in developing and driving forward an ambitious year-long arts programme encompassing painting, sculpture, music, drama and poetry. Poet Eavan Boland and playwright Marina Carr were writers-in-residence for the year. We organized high-profile classical music concerts, visual art exhibitions and ground-breaking scientific conferences.

Mary Robinson's election as President in 1990 had marked a moment of transition in Irish public life. It seemed to have the subtle effect of making it easier to espouse liberal causes. I asked if she would become a patron of the hospital – I thought having her associated with Holles Street would reinforce the message of change. She had had her children in Holles Street and kindly agreed. She was very generous with her time throughout the centenary year, in particular hosting a presidential dinner at the Royal Hospital Kilmainham.

During the centenary year we also commissioned a survey on women's health needs. Coordinated by the Economic and Social Research Institute, it was the largest survey of its kind in Ireland, and we intended that it should provide the framework for the development of women's healthcare strategies into the future. Three thousand women aged between eighteen and sixty gave their views on a range of issues, including pregnancy, menopause, family planning, breastfeeding, nutrition and social health.

On the clinical front, our centenary year also saw the return of Peter McParland from Canada as a fully trained fetal medicine specialist, and as master I was able to appoint him director of the service. His appointment meant that I was no longer carrying the service single-handedly, which reduced my clinical workload significantly.★

The year was rounded off with the publication of the hospital's centenary history. Social historian and publisher Tony Farmar wrote a vivid, meticulously researched account of the hospital's first hundred years.† Tony found that in 1894 one in ten infants died, and twice as many mothers died of childbirth as of tuberculosis. A century later, Ireland was one of the safest places in the world in which to have a baby. The National Maternity Hospital began as a tiny private charity in three dilapidated tenement houses looking after mothers from some of the worst slums in Europe. It was transformed by money from the Irish Hospitals Sweepstake in the 1930s, and by the 1990s it was one of the busiest maternity hospitals in Europe, and

---

★ The specialty thrived under Peter's leadership in the next couple of decades. By 2017 there were seven fetal medicine specialists on the consultant staff, and five midwife sonographers, providing a national service and receiving referrals from every unit in the country.

† Tony Farmar, *Holles Street 1894–1994: The National Maternity Hospital – A Centenary History* (Dublin: A & A Farmar, 1994). Tony, who was my brother-in-law, died in December 2017.

a focus of international interest in the development of obstetrics and gynaecology.

For me, the centenary year was exhilarating and at times exhausting, but very worthwhile. Women attending the hospital during the year enjoyed the buzz and excitement. The impact on staff morale and collegiality was exceptional – after the difficulties of the 1980s, the atmosphere was now positive, and a healthy pride in the institution flourished. And, crucially, the celebrations reawakened the public's affection for the hospital and reminded people of its significance to Dublin and Ireland.

No mother died during the course of pregnancy or in the postpartum period during 1994. Perhaps more than anything else, as I noted in the year's annual report, 'this clear fact represents perhaps the greatest single advance in the care of mothers in the first century of the hospital's activities. One hundred years ago one would have expected perhaps twenty-five mothers to have died during the course of pregnancy or soon afterwards. This great improvement is due to a combination of factors, not least the vast improvements in medical practice, particularly the availability of antibiotics, blood transfusion, and developments in anaesthesia.'

Similarly I noted the great improvement in perinatal mortality over the century. In 1894 – as Tony Farmar had recorded – one in every ten babies born at the hospital died shortly after birth or in the six weeks after. In 1994 the rate was 7.2 per thousand, meaning that 99.3 per cent of babies who weighed at least 500g at birth survived (excluding those with a fatal fetal abnormality for whom, sadly, nothing could be done). I was also happy to report in the centenary year that newborn intensive care was one of the most dramatic examples of improvements in medicine over the previous twenty years. The increased survival rate of small premature babies was enormously assisted by intensive nursing and medical care involving the use of increasingly sophisticated technology. (And in the twenty-five years since the centenary year, even more significant developments have taken place in neonatal intensive care, so that in 2019 babies born as prematurely as twenty-three weeks may survive.)

In 1995 more than 40 per cent of all women who delivered at Holles Street were first-time mothers, reflecting the declining size of families, and also giving rise to pressure on resources. First births are more difficult than subsequent ones: labour is longer and the Caesarean section rate is higher, resulting in longer bed-stay. First-time mothers also require more midwifery care to establish breast-feeding and help with care of the newborn baby. The epidural rate for first-time mothers was now 70 per cent. Thankfully, for the fourth year in a row, there was no maternal death, and the infant perinatal mortality rate was the lowest in the hospital's history.

There was an increase in the number of babies transferred into the neonatal unit from other hospitals, which I saw as a tribute to our growing national reputation. In 1995 I was encouraged to see also that the number of women referred to the gynaecology department increased by a huge 33 per cent over the previous year. I took it to mean that we were making significant progress in reassuring women, and the GPs who were referring them, about the hospital. Holles Street was now firmly set on a course of development and expansion.

While there were, sadly, three maternal deaths during the seven years of my mastership, two in my first year and one in my last, at the end of 1996 I was able to report the fifth year in a row with no maternal deaths. All departments of the hospital experienced increased activity. The number of babies born rose by over 8 per cent. A massive 45 per cent – 3,212 women – were first-time mothers, the largest percentage in the hospital's history.

I made my last annual report as master in 1997. At the very end of my term of office, in response to a request by the Department of Health, the three Dublin maternity hospitals presented our Strategic Review Report. Its focus was on the development of the services we provided, including our tertiary referral responsibilities, in a coherent and planned manner for the future. Between us we had seen a 21 per cent increase in the number of mothers delivered since 1994, and a remarkable 30 per cent increase in the number of first-time mothers, with all the implications for resources I have described. There was considerable pressure on beds, and midwifery staff, in particular, were increasingly stretched.

My relationship with the Department of Health was at times fractious. On several occasions during my years as master I was summoned to the Department and rebuked for spending more than the hospital's allocation. On one occasion the minister of the day, Brian Cowen, was present when I remarked that we couldn't provide the service to the women without the necessary resources and described it as a 'Pass Maths' equation, not a remark that endeared me to Department officials. In my final year as master, the leaden hand of the Department manifested itself yet again with its refusal to allow us to expand the facilities at the Merrion Wing, just as the VHI was announcing that it was recruiting 1,000 new members each week.

A favourite tactic of the Department – and a source of great frustration to me – was neither to acknowledge nor to reply to correspondence from the hospital. So, at the end of my mastership, I wrote to one of the assistant secretaries and requested that my successor be at least given the courtesy of a reply to any letter he might write to the Department. Needless to say, I got no reply.

Though I had always had great belief in the mastership system, my conclusion at the end of my term was that as a method of running a maternity hospital it could not be bettered – primarily, because a doctor has a better understanding of the real 'business' of a maternity hospital than any non-medic could ever have. No matter how hardworking or well intentioned or competent, it is impossible for a non-medic truly to understand the nature of how a hospital works. They are not present at doctor–patient interactions, at overloaded clinics, at complicated deliveries at four o'clock in the morning, at meetings with bereaved parents or spouses, trying to explain the inexplicable. I also concluded that it was critically important that the master should continue in clinical practice, as otherwise there would be a danger of becoming detached from the real purpose of the hospital, the care of women, and every activity had to remain subservient to this.

I found my years as master to be an enormously rewarding experience and one I enjoyed immensely. I was, however, hugely relieved to pass the baton to Declan Keane and relinquish the twenty-four hours a day, seven days a week, responsibility. Having fulfilled my professional life's ambition, I left the hospital on 31 December 1997, knowing that when I next walked back through its doors it would no longer be as master. The mastership ends on the stroke of midnight on New Year's Eve, and Frances and I had a welcome glass of champagne to celebrate my freedom. I looked forward to a more relaxed life.

6.   An obstetrician's working week

When leaving the mastership behind I might have told myself – and assured my family – that now I was returning to a somewhat easier pace of life, but life as a working obstetrician is not relaxed. Babies are born at all hours of the day and night, so on top of doing the day job there was always the ever-present likelihood of having to go back to the hospital during the night.

Typically, on an average working day, I arrived into my office at 7.30 a.m., put on a white coat and went into the 'Res', the doctor's residence, for coffee, to pick up post and catch up with colleagues. The juniors who had been on-duty through the night were usually gathered there, exhausted and resuscitating themselves with coffee and a bowl of cereal. The busyness of the night was often reflected in the number of half-eaten pizzas and half-empty coffee cups on the table indicating interrupted meals. We would chat about their night and any interesting or difficult cases they had dealt with.

If I was on-duty for the hospital that day, I would go next to the delivery ward to meet the midwife in charge, and, together with the registrar, we would do a round of the labour ward, meeting each woman, and usually her partner. The purpose of the ward round was not to 'interfere' in the conduct of the labours being managed by the midwives but to make myself aware of what was happening, since, as the consultant on-duty, I was ultimately responsible. If one of the midwives called me in to deal with an emergency or complicated delivery, I would know who the patient was and, if I needed to become involved in the delivery, I would not be a stranger to the woman.

A complicated clinical scenario might be a woman having a vaginal breech delivery (where the baby reverses out of the birth canal bottom first instead of coming head first) for the second of a pair of twins. The danger is that the baby's head may get stuck, which can cause a fatal brain haemorrhage, or oxygen deprivation, which can cause disability. Vaginal breech delivery is very unusual nowadays, as most babies in that position are delivered by Caesarean section. In consequence the skill of delivering a breech baby vaginally is being lost. I occasionally saw a woman in the antenatal clinic who wished to attempt a vaginal breech delivery, but I was unable to facilitate her because I couldn't guarantee that someone would be on-duty who had the experience to perform the delivery – a sad state of affairs but the reality of modern obstetrics as the Caesarean section rate continues to increase. All I could say to her was that if there was a doctor present in the hospital who was comfortable with the procedure when she was about to deliver, we would give her that option, of course, but it could not be guaranteed. If no one was available she would have to have an emergency Caesarean section.

After visiting the labour ward I would go to my antenatal clinic. I had one morning and one afternoon clinic each week. As there were up to 100 women attending, it was obviously impossible for me to see each woman individually. There were five rooms, or cubicles, and there were a registrar and senior house officer to assist, as well as a midwife running her* own clinic in one of the cubicles. I saw each woman on her first visit and, as I often told women who asked, after that first visit seeing the midwife was usually at least as good as if not better than seeing me or another obstetrician. Women seeing the same midwife on their visits could build up a relationship with her.

The antenatal clinic was always a lively and interesting place and the hours flew by. It was incredibly busy, with phones ringing, junior doctors being bleeped to attend to a patient on a postnatal ward (there weren't enough juniors to have one dedicated to the postnatal ward), medical students being taught the rudiments of antenatal care, blood and other laboratory results having to be checked, patients having to be phoned with results of tests, charts of previous pregnancies needing to be reviewed and ongoing paperwork around everything else – forms to be signed for air travel or maternity leave, or letters needing to be handwritten† for employers when a patient needed time off work because of a complication of pregnancy.

---

* For the vast majority of my working life the midwives I worked with were female. Of course, there are excellent male midwives as well. For simplicity I refer to midwives as female throughout the book.

† Doctors in the public health system do not have any personal secretarial support, which is a factor in the recruitment of doctors. Any paperwork that needs doing

As the years went on the range of nationalities attending the ante-natal clinics broadened remarkably. In the late 1990s and early 2000s there were quite a number of Nigerian patients, often only arriving in the country in the late stages of pregnancy and with no medical records. At the time any child born in Ireland was entitled to Irish, and therefore European, citizenship and the Rotunda and the Coombe had a similar experience. In the years that followed we saw women from virtually every country in the world. Language was occasionally a problem, and if things were complicated we had to get a translator to attend with the woman. The patient profile today reflects the welcome diversity of modern Ireland.

One morning a week I had an operating theatre list that started at 8 a.m. The evening before, I would go to the ward and see the women due for major surgery the next day, hysterectomy, for example, and discuss the procedure with them and answer any questions they might have. Informed consent was an important part of the pre-operative discussion. This consisted of explaining to the woman what the operation involved and what could go wrong. Sometimes informing patients of possible complications had the counterproductive effect of making them more nervous than they needed to be. Usually, however, women were reassured that the likelihood of a serious complication was rare.

Younger women having hysterectomies might also have to consider whether their ovaries should be removed or not. If the ovaries were taken out, the menopause began almost immediately because the production of oestrogen ceased, but on the positive side the chances of developing ovarian cancer were reduced to almost zero. Of course, we would have teased this out in advance in clinic visits – but, understandably, the prospect of being plunged into an early and sudden menopause was daunting. A doctor does not tell a woman what she should do; rather we give her all the relevant information and answer her questions as fully as possible so that she can make an informed decision.

After arriving in the theatre on the morning of surgery I changed

---

has to be done on the fly – in a case like this, as part of the consultation, or some-how fitted in around seeing patients.

into my first set of blue scrubs for the day (as they generally became blood-stained during the course of surgery, there would be a few changes throughout the day) and a pair of wooden clogs (when you're standing for many hours clogs are more supportive). Other members of the team were present, including anaesthesiologists, theatre nursing staff and junior doctors.

The operating list comprised major cases, like hysterectomies or planned Caesarean sections, and minor cases such as miscarriages or laparoscopies (inspecting the pelvis with a telescope-like instrument under general anaesthetic). Two operating theatres were active during the list, and when not operating, or assisting, I, like my consultant colleagues, would go between the two to supervise surgery (trainees learn by performing surgery under supervision – that's how I and all consultants learned).

Because the hospital was so busy there would inevitably be interruptions to the list of scheduled procedures because of emergency Caesareans coming from the labour ward. Some emergencies were more urgent than others – for example, a Caesarean section for fetal distress where the baby is showing signs of lack of oxygen is more urgent than one for a slow or prolonged labour, although both are classified as emergencies. There were also gynaecological emergencies such as ectopic pregnancies or women bleeding heavily following a miscarriage.

From a surgeon's point of view most surgery is rather mundane, so when things go wrong it really stands out in the memory. The ability to combine a sense of urgency with clarity and calmness, to assess and reassess what is often a rapidly evolving situation, while all the time adrenaline is pumping through you, is a real test of your capacity as a surgeon.

One February evening in 2012 I was chatting with colleagues in the operating theatres' coffee room after a ward round, when I was called urgently to an emergency in one of the theatres. A registrar performing an emergency Caesarean section for fetal distress had opened the patient's abdomen and found that all he could see was blood. I wasn't operating that day but I changed, got scrubbed up, and put on a sterile operating gown and gloves as quickly as possible. The first task was to deliver the baby, a boy, and hand him to the paediatricians. Because it was an emergency operation and no other theatre was available, we were working in a small operating theatre normally used for minor procedures. There wasn't room to accommodate the resuscitation equipment for the paediatricians so they took the baby away.

I thought the source of the bleeding might be a rupture or a tear in the uterus. On inspection this wasn't the case, however. To explore the abdomen and find the source of the bleeding, I immediately extended the incision vertically towards the patient's chest. The original incision had been a standard one for Caesarean section across the lower abdomen in the 'bikini line'.

Around me the team sprang into action. The anaesthesiologist ordered blood for transfusion. A second anaesthesiologist came to help monitor the patient's vital signs. Together they inserted additional intravenous lines to help with resuscitation. Porters were dispatched to the laboratory with blood samples for urgent testing and to bring blood back for transfusion. A nurse kept track of the amount of blood lost (torrential initially) and the amount of fluids infused. While all this was going on, I was trying to locate the source of the bleeding. The number of staff in the room grew from the usual four to around ten.

The bleeding was coming from the upper abdomen, and as the registrar continued to suck out blood and apply pressure with large swabs I could see that the source of the bleeding was the splenic artery, a large artery under the diaphragm that had ruptured. This was a potentially fatal complication for the mother; it normally carries with it a 75 per cent mortality rate for the mother and a 95 per cent fatality rate for the baby (though in this case a living baby had been delivered).

By this time other consultant colleagues had arrived to help. I asked one of them to phone the vascular surgery team in St Vincent's Hospital to request their assistance. (Vascular surgeons specialize in procedures related to arteries and veins.) While we waited for their arrival all I could do was staunch the flow of blood by keeping my fist pressed hard against several large swabs over the rupture.

Meanwhile, the team from St Vincent's – surgeon Mary Barry and a theatre nurse with their specialist equipment – were on their way in a taxi, their journey delayed because Ireland and the Czech Republic were playing in a friendly international at the nearby Aviva Stadium.

While the wait was no more than thirty minutes, it felt like hours. The anaesthesiologists were continually transfusing blood and monitoring the patient's condition. The laboratory staff were giving us the results of the blood tests for haemoglobin and blood clotting factors. The woman's vital signs remained stable but when so much blood is lost so quickly there is a risk of organ failure and death.

I handed over to Mary Barry, and over the course of two hours she sealed off the rupture and the patient was stabilized and her life saved. She was transferred to the intensive care unit at St Vincent's. The baby survived but unfortunately had suffered from lack of oxygen for some minutes, which resulted in a degree of disability.

By an extraordinary coincidence the patient was actually in Holles Street attending a routine antenatal clinic that afternoon when she suddenly felt unwell. This undoubtedly saved her life and that of her baby. A delay in getting her to theatre would almost certainly have been fatal for both. She and her partner understood what had happened to her and were naturally extremely relieved and grateful for how events that afternoon and evening transpired.

Cases like this illustrate the benefits of co-locating maternity and general hospitals to provide access to intensive care and specialist teams. Although in this particular case the outcome would have been no different had we been on the St Vincent's campus, the conditions were less than ideal and there was a delay in the arrival of the specialist surgeon.

The time around surgery is extremely stressful for patients and can cause them to act out of character. One Thursday morning in February 2006 I was preparing to perform a hysterectomy when I took a phone call to inform me that my mother had died. She was ninety-three and, although she had been unwell for some time, her death still came as a shock and a great sadness. I went to the patient to apologize and explain why I would not be able to do her operation. She thought this unreasonable on my part. I offered her the choice of rescheduling with me or I could arrange someone else to do it later that day, but she wasn't for turning. I had to explain to her, in the nicest possible way, that I wouldn't be operating any further that day as my concentration, for reasons obvious to me at least, wouldn't be the best. I gave her the benefit of the doubt and put her behaviour down to anxiety. I always tried to help trainees to understand that people under stress can sometimes act unreasonably and be aggressive but that they should never take it personally; the job of the professional is to 'suck it up' and remember that stress and worry about surgery or illness may be responsible for the behaviour.

One afternoon a week I had a colposcopy clinic. Colposcopy is the examination of the cervix with a high-powered binocular-type instrument. It is performed to follow up on an abnormal smear test picked up in a screening programme.

Cervical smears are not designed to detect cancer. They are designed to detect and diagnose abnormalities in the cervix that might develop into a cancer if left untreated. Most benign abnormalities can be treated immediately at the time of colposcopy.

Women attending the clinic were often extremely anxious because they feared that an abnormal smear might mean that they had cancer. So the most important thing to say during the examination was 'you don't have cancer.' Women's relief on hearing those words was palpable. A fair amount of my time during the consultation was spent reassuring patients that their condition was benign, educating them about the nature of changes in the cervix, and explaining that if they adhered to the treatment plan the chances of developing cancer, while not zero, were extremely low. Those who ended up having to attend the clinic on a regular basis tended to be less anxious as they developed a better understanding of the process.

Occasionally, however, a woman presented with an abnormality and the colposcopic exam was suspicious. A biopsy would then be performed. The woman was phoned with the result if the result was benign or asked to come in for a discussion if it wasn't. I would explain to the woman what the diagnosis was – cancer of the cervix – and what the next steps were going to be.

Although most women coming in for a conversation about a biopsy suspected the worst, I could see how the news that they had cancer still hit them like a thunderbolt. Often a diagnosis like this caused a patient to go into a sort of daze of incomprehension. I always made sure to have a nurse with me for these conversations to support the patient and arrange the next steps – usually a CT scan and an appointment with a cancer specialist. Frightening as a cancer diagnosis is, women with early, and limited, cervical cancer can be treated relatively conservatively and even go on to have successful pregnancies if they wish.

★

The Tuesday morning fetal medicine conference was one of the highlights of the week. This brought together fetal medicine specialists, neonatal paediatricians, paediatric cardiologists, pathologists, geneticists, and paediatric surgeons from Temple Street and Crumlin Children's Hospitals, to discuss cases that had been seen by the fetal medicine specialists, often having been referred from various hospitals around the country when some fetal abnormality had been diagnosed on ultrasound.

We discussed possible treatments. These might include intrauterine surgery on a fetus, such as draining a collection of fluid around the lungs, or laser surgery to treat twin-to-twin transfusion syndrome (the situation described in the Dunne case, where one twin loses blood and the other receives it, and both are seriously compromised). It is a very serious condition. This surgery would be performed in a collaboration between NMH and Rotunda fetal medicine specialists.

In the conference the relevant specialists would develop a plan of management and afterwards hold a clinic where the parents of the affected fetus would be counselled regarding prognosis and possible treatment options. Before talking to the parents an optimal delivery plan would be worked out. This often generated lively discussion about the relative merits of a planned Caesarean, induction of labour or allowing spontaneous labour. Paediatricians tended to prefer Caesareans because they could then anticipate the time of delivery. With induced births, the time of delivery couldn't be predicted and it might be in the middle of the night, which was not ideal if a full team of paediatricians was required at the birth or the baby required urgent transfer to Temple Street or Crumlin.

If the prognosis was hopeless, or if there was no great urgency about transfer to a paediatric hospital, the mothers were encouraged to deliver in their own local hospitals. Some were reluctant to return to their referring hospital – understandably they wanted to remain in a hospital with a high level of expertise even if we reassured them that the birth would be normal or no immediate interventions would be needed, or if we told them that, tragically, their baby would not survive birth even with all of our expertise and experience. Sometimes the referring hospital was reluctant to take back the patient, citing unfamiliarity with the relevant condition or lack of appropriately skilled consultant paediatric staff. Given the level of pressure on resources in maternity units around the country, they were probably glad to have one fewer birth to manage, particularly if it was one where there was a complication with the baby's health. Of course, the more such births ended up happening in tertiary hospitals like the NMH, the less experience colleagues gained in the smaller units around the country.

Occasionally the conference was given over to a lecture from a colleague with some specialized interest. I can recall Michael Early, a consultant paediatric plastic surgeon, giving a fascinating lecture, with his own illustrations, on the vastly improved surgical treatment of cleft lip and palate. Nowadays the surgery is so good that it is often impossible to tell it has been done. Another favourite was Dr William Reardon, who lectured us on genetic developments, amply illustrated by puzzles he had solved that had eluded others – he was a man who clearly took great pleasure in his work and his talks were always entertaining and informative.

Obstetrics is not the profession for anyone who wants to work routine hours. Night and weekend duty are burdens every obstetrician lives with and of course these are on top of a regular day or week's work. Lunch is all too often an apple grabbed on the move. In later years when my phone could track my steps, I found I could easily exceed my 10,000 steps per day, much of it spent running up and down the back stairs in Holles Street between the labour ward, the operating theatre and my office. On nights when I was on call, prior to going home around 6.30 or 7 p.m., I would review what was happening in the labour ward by doing a round of all the women there, with the senior midwife and registrar. I would then check for any potential problems in the antenatal ward, the gynae ward where post-operative patients were recuperating, and finally the operating theatre to see if any surgery was being performed.

At home I would wait for the inevitable phone calls from the registrar on-duty about developing problems in the labour ward. Usually the calls were to make a decision about whether or not to do a Caesarean section. In the course of a night on-duty I would often make one or more trips into the hospital if there were particularly complicated deliveries or Caesarean sections.

Weekends on call began on Friday morning and lasted until

Monday morning when I went back into the hospital to commence a normal working week. It was not unusual to go into the hospital several times a day over the weekend for a combination of ward rounds in an attempt to anticipate problems and deal with them early, and to catch up on paperwork. And, of course, right through the weekend there would be calls at night – the frequency of these being dependent on the seniority and experience of the registrar on-duty, or if a particularly complicated case arose.

Being on call meant that weekends would have to be spent close to home and the hospital. Family and friends grew used to my sudden disappearances in the middle of meals or watching movies. Sometimes I would arrive back an hour later and rejoin the occasion. Other times I would come back to a dark and silent house with everyone having long gone to bed. There was no question of sailing in Dublin Bay but gardening proved to be a good hobby. Luckily, I live close enough to Holles Street so that at night – with no traffic on the roads (and occasionally breaking a red light if the situation was particularly urgent) – I could be in the operating theatre within ten minutes of getting a phone call. Daylight hours were not so simple. On one occasion I was at a Christmas lunch at a restaurant on Stephen's Green when I was called to an emergency at the hospital. I was edging into the Christmas traffic, easing through a red light, when a garda motorcycle drew alongside me and in that typical garda way – where they ask you a question but it's really an accusation – the officer asked me if I realized that I was breaking a red light. No doubt he suspected I was a Christmas reveller who'd had a glass of wine too many over lunch. However, when I explained I was on my way to Holles Street for an emergency he immediately switched on his siren and provided an escort to the hospital. I was a bit mortified but it was one of those moments that brought home to me the significance of the work – everyone knows what's at stake when you explain an obstetric emergency and everyone wants to help. The privilege of spending one's life doing work of this nature – looking after women at the most important moments in their lives – outweighs the long hours, the unpredictability and the constant underlying pressure. Having a sense of purpose like that is a gift that I never underestimated.

PART II

7.   Savita

Savita Andanappa Yalagi was born in the southern Indian city of Bagalkot in 1981. She was the third child and only daughter of Andanappa and Akhmedevi Yalagi. In 2008 she married Praveen Halappanavar, an engineer at Boston Scientific in Galway. July 2012 was a good month for the young couple. Savita had qualified as a dentist outside Europe, and had sat the Irish Dental Council examinations so that she could practise in Ireland; in July she was granted her licence. And later in the month they were delighted to find out that Savita was pregnant. Their baby was due at the end of March 2013.

On 11 October Savita had a routine antenatal visit at University Hospital Galway, when her blood pressure, weight, urine, and blood tests were all normal. She was noted to have suffered from lower back pain for some years that recently had got worse, and she was referred to a physiotherapist, whom she saw the following week.

Ten days later, on Sunday, 21 October, she returned to the hospital because of back pain. Following assessment she was discharged home, as there was nothing obviously wrong with the pregnancy at that point. Later on Sunday she went back to the hospital because she could feel a sensation of pressure in her vagina. The doctor who examined her felt that her cervix was dilating, and she was admitted for further observation. Later that evening the waters around the baby ruptured. As a medical professional herself, she understood the implications of her situation – that at seventeen weeks the outlook for her baby was dismal.

The couple were told that Savita's cervix was fully dilated, amniotic fluid was leaking, and 'unfortunately the baby wouldn't survive.' Afterwards Praveen Halappanavar said that his wife asked several times over three days for the pregnancy to be terminated. 'Savita was really in agony . . . She was very upset, but she accepted she was losing the baby. When the consultant came on the ward rounds [the morning after she was admitted to hospital] Savita asked if they could not save the baby could they induce to end the pregnancy. The consultant said, "As long as there is a fetal heartbeat we can't do anything." '

It was reported that a midwife told Savita that 'This is a Catholic country' in response to her requests for a termination. Savita, a Hindu, told hospital staff, 'I am neither Irish nor Catholic,' but she was once more told there was nothing they could do. Two days later she was critically ill and had miscarried her daughter. By the evening of her fourth day in hospital, she was in intensive care. Three days later Savita was dead.

The story broke in the round-up of the next day's newspapers on Vincent Browne's late-night TV show on 13 November. Under the headline 'Woman "Denied a Termination" Dies in Hospital', Kitty Holland's story was on the front page of the *Irish Times*. The story was accompanied by a photograph of a smiling Savita, an image that would become iconic.

Savita's death was the principal item in the Order of Business in both the Dáil and the Seanad on 14 November. The following day Praveen spoke from India to Sean O'Rourke on RTÉ's *News at One*. He told the story of his wife's last days and hours with courage and composure.

In her book *Savita: The Tragedy That Shook a Nation* Kitty Holland described how the *Irish Times* story went viral in a matter of hours, dominating Irish media and, to her initial surprise, attracting attention from CNN, the BBC World Service, Channel 4 News, Sky News, the *Telegraph*, the *Guardian*, France 24, Al Jazeera and *El País* among others.*

In India the story elicited shock and anger. The indiatimes.com website ran the headline 'Ireland Murders Indian Dentist'. There were protests outside the Irish Embassy in Delhi, and in towns and cities in Karnataka. Abortion had been decriminalized in India in 1971, and Savita's friends and family simply could not understand why, as they saw it, basic medical treatment was denied to her in a modern European country. Savita's mother told Indian television that '[I]n an attempt to save a four-month-old-fetus, they killed my thirty-year-old daughter. How is that fair, you tell me?' Her father

---

*Kitty Holland, *Savita: The Tragedy That Shook a Nation* (Dublin and London: Transworld Ireland, 2013), 82–3.

was reported as telling the *Times of India* that '[I]f the Irish law on abortion is changed, I would think my daughter has been sacrificed for a good cause.'

I first became aware of the story when my phone started to beep during my usual Wednesday morning antenatal clinic in Holles Street. I hadn't seen the paper or heard the morning news, a not unusual experience for hospital doctors on busy clinic or theatre days. It was immediately apparent to me from the level of media interest that people were deeply affected by Savita's death. That evening in Dublin about 2,000 people, mainly women, gathered outside the Dáil. Kildare Street was closed, as those present sat down in the street and observed silence in memory of Savita. My wife Jane,* who was there, thought the mood was one of deep shock and upset.

RTÉ Radio 1's *Morning Ireland* asked me to come on the following day. By then, and beyond my practice in Holles Street, I was very familiar with the fault-line where clinical practice intersected with the law on termination. The 1992 Supreme Court judgment on the X case was the law of the state. The X case arose when the attorney general sought an interim High Court injunction to prevent a pregnant fourteen-year-old girl, a rape victim, from travelling to the UK for an abortion. The girl was already in the UK so her parents brought her back to Dublin, at which point the High Court injunction was made permanent. The family appealed the decision to the Supreme Court, and by a four to one majority the court decided that the girl, Miss X, had a right to travel for an abortion. But the court went further. In arguing X's case in the High Court her counsel had presented evidence that she was suicidal. The Supreme Court held that if it was established as a matter of probability that there was a real and substantial risk to the life, as distinct from the health, of the mother, and that this real and substantial risk could be averted only by the termination of her pregnancy, such a termination was lawful. In other words, the X case judgment established a right to abortion *in Ireland*. Crucially, however, there were no guidelines in existence as to how this real and substantial risk to the mother's life could be quantified.

* Sadly, my marriage to Frances had broken up in 2001. Some years later I met Jane Mahony and we married in 2011.

Moreover, the Offences Against the Person Act 1861 remained in force, and so any doctor who unlawfully procured an abortion could face life in prison with hard labour. The Supreme Court set down general principles in the judgment, and made it clear that it was the job of the Oireachtas to legislate. Over two decades successive governments failed to do so.

In December 2009 the European Court of Human Rights (ECHR) ruled that there had been a violation by the state of the rights of a woman, named as C, under Article 8 of the Convention for the Protection of Human Rights and Fundamental Freedoms. The ECHR held that there was no accessible and effective procedure to enable C to establish if she had the right to a lawful termination of pregnancy in Ireland. The judgment noted the 'significant chilling effect' of existing Irish legislation.

Earlier in 2012 the Minister for Health, James Reilly, had invited me to sit on an expert group chaired by Mr Justice Sean Ryan. We were tasked with providing a series of options on how to implement the X judgment in the light of the ECHR ruling. By an extraordinary coincidence, our report was delivered to the government on the evening of Tuesday, 13 November, the day before the story of Savita's death was published in the *Irish Times*.

On *Morning Ireland* Rachael English asked me if doctors in Ireland were 'flying blind' when trying to determine when a termination of pregnancy was legal in Ireland. I explained how in certain circumstances we were very clear about what to do. These might include the treatment of a woman with very high blood pressure who was liable to have seizures that might result in blindness or death. Another example might be where a woman haemorrhaged severely at sixteen or eighteen weeks, and failure to terminate the pregnancy would mean her bleeding to death. The problem was in the grey areas where we did not have certainty, but had to proceed on the basis of probability. If we got it wrong, we were, I explained, 'committing a criminal offence as the law stands' and the consequences would be very grave. The problem, of course, is that as the practice of medicine is full of probabilities, certainty is rarely attainable.

I could not comment in the interview on a particular case, and in any event had no knowledge at that point of what had happened to Savita apart from what had been reported in the newspapers. Rachael

English asked me if I had encountered similar cases. I told her that 'If there are no signs of infection, then we are prohibited [from terminating a pregnancy] by the law of the land.' I said that as doctors we wanted to be able to practise medicine in a safe environment legally, but 'the current situation is like the Sword of Damocles hanging over us. If we do something with a good intention, but it turns out to be illegal, the consequences are extremely serious for medical practitioners.' Doctors and women needed the threat of criminality removed, I said, and legislators needed to do their duty to protect the people who were looking after the state's citizens.

My intention was to turn the focus to the vacuum that had existed since the X case. In my view, the failure to legislate in the two decades was a disgrace, and entirely the responsibility of our legislators. It seemed outrageous that politicians could shirk such important legislation, while trumpeting their success in getting potholes in their local constituency filled or securing passports for constituents.

In the following days I was contacted by media organizations around the world. Many journalists picked up my Sword of Damocles image as a useful metaphor for the precarious and delicate situation that the Eighth Amendment forced on Irish obstetricians.

Over the next several weeks Savita's story dominated the news. I could see a division in public opinion about the implications of the case based on whether people described themselves as 'pro-life' or not. Many who called themselves pro-life maintained that Savita's death had nothing to do with the Eighth Amendment, but must have been due to clinical mismanagement during her time in UHG.

Describing oneself as pro-life has always seemed to me to be either a cynical or an unthinking attempt to occupy the moral high ground while demonstrating little or no empathy with fellow human beings who are mothers, sisters, friends and colleagues. Indeed, in my practice I had met couples who self-described as ardently pro-life, but who changed their minds and proceeded with termination when confronted with the painful reality of a pregnancy that was not going to result in a live baby due to a fatal fetal abnormality. In the context of the death of a young, pregnant woman, the use of the term seemed offensive.

The Taoiseach, Enda Kenny, and Fianna Fáil leader Micheál Martin agreed that no conclusions should be reached until the results of the various inquiries were available for scrutiny. Since either Fianna Fáil or Fine Gael had been the main party of government for the entire time since the Supreme Court had criticized the Oireachtas for not legislating for the X case, neither party would accept responsibility for that failure. And it seemed that yet again neither party had any enthusiasm for dealing with such a political hot potato. But as public outrage mounted, doing nothing was no longer an option.

It became clear that some Fine Gael TDs who were on the record as holding anti-abortion views had been shaken by Savita's death. The young Wicklow TD Simon Harris said: 'In the past I've said I didn't see the need to legislate. Let me assure you today I am reconsidering. There can be no grey areas.' Meanwhile Charlie Flanagan, chair of Fine Gael's Parliamentary Party, said: 'I really do feel for the family of Savita. I read comments attributed to Praveen, as a husband and a partner. And I mean, I ask myself, what would I do in such circumstances? How would I wish matters might proceed in such circumstances? And I say that as a public representative, as a father of two daughters and as a husband. And I just think that women's lives come before any ideology and must be protected primarily.'

Just before Christmas 2012, the coroner for the West Galway district, Dr Ciaran McLoughlin, asked if I would assist the inquest to be held the following April as his expert witness. During phone calls over the next several weeks he indicated that he wanted me to comment on the possible influence of the law on Savita's care.

I was sent Savita's full medical records and went through them line by line, word by word, measurement by measurement. As an expert medical witness, you work on fact and science, not conjecture or emotion. Despite the media coverage, I could not make any assumptions until I had forensically analysed her medical records.

On the morning of 17 April, a cold, wet Wednesday, I sat in a coroner's court in Galway to begin giving my evidence on Savita Halappanavar's death. How I had approached it was to visualize the various stages of Savita's course in hospital as a kind of analogue Geiger counter, where the needle on the dial moved from safe levels on the left-hand side, to danger and death on the right. The question that would move the needle, as I observed in my report to the inquest, was: 'At any given point was there a real and substantial risk of death for Ms Halappanavar which could only be averted by termination of the pregnancy?' Would it be possible to identify the moment when a termination was legal in Ireland, had the doctors identified that moment or not, and at the appropriate time or not?

I began my evidence with an outline of sepsis in pregnancy, the leading cause of maternal death in the UK, though with a relatively low mortality rate of 1 in 100,000 pregnancies in the UK. Figures for Ireland were similar: for example, in the NMH in the previous twenty-five years, over 210,000 women had given birth and there had been two maternal deaths from sepsis, one of which was at a gestation similar to Savita's and had occurred during my mastership. So, while fortunately death and serious illness from pregnancy-related sepsis are still rare, it means that many healthcare workers have never seen a case, so awareness and the index of suspicion are low.

Sepsis is a serious complication of an infection. Without quick and effective treatment it can progress to multi-organ failure and death. What is called the 'fulminating' nature of sepsis, i.e., abrupt and severe onset or deterioration, is surprising and shocking when it happens. In evidence earlier in the inquest one of the midwives who nursed Savita said that she had never seen anyone 'get so sick so quickly'.

I prepared a detailed chronology of Savita's course in UHG. At intervals, with the mental dial in mind, I noted whether or not at each of those given points the treatment Savita received was appropriate and whether or not her life was in danger.

On Sunday, 21 October 2012, Savita was experiencing worsening back pain and went to the UHG maternity unit to get checked. She was seventeen weeks pregnant. Up to this point her pregnancy had been normal and uncomplicated. At the hospital no specific cause for the pain was found, and, because Savita had a history of back pain going back nine years and was already seeing a physiotherapist about it, the SHO on-duty felt able to reassure her, give her painkillers and discharge her home. My comment to the inquest noted that her 'presentation at this point was typical of what happens commonly in the early stages of a pregnancy. The fact that Ms Halappanavar had a history of back pain was taken into account. Her management at this time was entirely appropriate.'

Later that afternoon, however, Savita went to the bathroom and felt 'something coming down', and she said she had 'pushed a leg back in'. Praveen brought her straight back to the hospital. The SHO who had seen her in the morning called the registrar on-duty. On examination it transpired that the membranes had prolapsed through the cervix and were bulging into the vagina. The membranes, like clingfilm, form the (amniotic) fluid-filled sac within which the baby develops during pregnancy and also prevent infection from ascending into the sac. The cervix, or neck of the uterus, is normally closed tightly during the pregnancy and keeps the membranes and sac within the uterus. For the membranes to prolapse into the vagina, the cervix must have opened enough to allow the membranes to bulge through.

The doctor who examined Savita was unable to feel the cervix, as the sac was in the way, and he, quite correctly, didn't want to perform a vigorous examination that might have ruptured the sac. Her pain was said to be 'unbearable', and she was noted to be distressed. She was given pethidine for the pain. It was documented that she had an 'inevitable/impending pregnancy loss' and that a stitch in the cervix was not appropriate. She was admitted to UHG 'with a plan to await events'.

The doctor gave the couple the sad news that at seventeen weeks there was no chance of survival for the baby if born. Savita's blood pressure, pulse and temperature were all normal at this time.

Savita was admitted to St Monica's Ward, and among the blood tests performed was a full blood count, which, among other measurements, counts the white blood cells. An abnormally high white blood cell count may indicate an infection. If a woman is not pregnant, the upper limit of normal is 10; in pregnancy, the upper limit ranges from 14 to 16. When Savita had first attended UHG earlier in the month, her count was 11.4, consistent with pregnancy. The white cell count taken on the Sunday returned a result of 16.9, and, although the results were available from the laboratory within a couple of hours, they were not read by the medical staff until days later.

My report observed that at her return to UHG 'it was clear that there was a major problem with the pregnancy and it appeared very probable she would miscarry. The full blood count taken after admission showed an elevated white cell count with a neutrophil account also elevated. This suggested the possibility of an infection. The report does not appear to have been incorporated into the notes and neither was it repeated. The site of a possible infection, however, was not clear. There were no other signs of infection. At this time, 21 October, there was nothing to indicate that Ms Halappanavar's life was in danger.' There was no discussion of termination, and Savita did not request one.

Savita did not appear to have any problems in the early part of Sunday evening. Her vital signs were normal, she was not in pain, and she declined any pain relief. At half past midnight she went to the bathroom and vomited. At the same time the membranes ruptured and amniotic fluid flowed out. A nurse helped her back into bed and noted that she was 'feeling better' without any complaints of pain, though she was very anxious. There was some light bleeding overnight.

On the ward round the next morning, Monday, 22 October, Savita was seen by the consultant obstetrician, Dr Katherine Astbury. Her history was recorded and she was noted to be 'bleeding like a period'. The plan of management was that she would have a scan for the presence or absence of the fetal heart and 'await events'. Savita's blood pressure, pulse and temperature were all normal. An antibiotic, erythromycin, was prescribed in accordance with standard international practice to minimize the risk of infection ascending into the uterus. The survival rate for the fetus following rupture of membranes at seventeen weeks is low, at approximately 10 per cent.

Dr Astbury subsequently said that had she known about the white cell count of 16.9 on the Sunday she would have arranged to repeat it on the Tuesday. However, the Royal College of Obstetricians and Gynaecologists (RCOG) guideline on the management of rupture of membranes in situations such as this states that '[I]t is not necessary to carry out weekly maternal full blood count or c-reactive protein because the sensitivity of these tests in the detection of intrauterine infection is low.' Thus, it was not a deficiency in Savita's care not to have repeated the white cell count. RCOG guidelines are used extensively internationally and virtually all consultant obstetricians in Ireland are members of the RCOG.

After the scan on the Monday, Savita asked to be delivered; in other words she asked for a termination of pregnancy. She understood fully that the prospect of survival for the baby was poor, and she wanted to get it over with. It was explained to her that this wasn't possible because there was still a fetal heartbeat present and termination wasn't legal unless her life was at risk. In the course of explaining this to her, a nurse said: 'This is a Catholic country.' In conversation with the nurse Savita had mentioned the Hindu faith and how in India there wouldn't be any hesitation in acceding to her wish, and she couldn't understand why the same didn't apply in Ireland. In her evidence to the inquest the nurse made it clear that in saying this she was trying to help Savita understand the context in which a termination was not possible.

During the Monday, Savita's temperature was normal on five occasions, and her pulse and blood pressure readings gave no cause for concern. I observed that the drug administration chart suggested that the first dose of the antibiotic that had been prescribed by Dr Astbury on Monday morning was not given until the next day, Tuesday, but that during Monday, 22 October, Savita 'remained stable and there was no evidence of infection'. 'There was nothing to indicate that Ms Halappanavar's life was in danger at this time.' Despite Savita's request for a termination, the law did not permit it on the Monday.

On the morning of Tuesday, 23 October, Savita's blood pressure was 100/65, pulse 84 and temperature 37.1, all normal. During the morning ward round Savita asked again about receiving medication to precipitate the impending miscarriage, i.e., to terminate the pregnancy. The legal situation in the country with regard to termination of pregnancy was explained to her again by Dr Astbury. Savita was very upset by this. A scan later that morning confirmed the presence of a fetal heartbeat. At noon, the fetal heart was checked for once more with a Doppler ultrasound scanner, but it was noted that this upset Savita, who requested that the heartbeat not be checked again. (Of course, even though it distressed her, staff would have had to disregard Savita's wishes about this.)

There was some bleeding during the day, which made the prospect of spontaneous miscarriage more likely, but there were no contractions and so the pregnancy continued. Temperature and blood pressure remained normal throughout the day, but the pulse rate remained above 100 from 2.45 p.m. onwards. The increase in pulse rate probably indicated the initial development of the infection that would result in her death. However, at no stage during the day was there a threat to her life that could be averted only by termination of pregnancy. I gave evidence therefore that '[T]ermination of pregnancy was not a practical, legal, proposition on the 23rd.'

Late on the Tuesday evening a nurse asked a doctor to review Savita, as she was feeling weak. Her blood pressure was noted to be stable and her heart-rate in the 90–100 range since admission. The unit was extremely busy that night with some very ill patients, and it was 1 a.m. on Wednesday, the 24th, by the time he got to the ward. Savita was asleep and so he didn't want to wake her up to ask her how she was feeling. This was a reasonable response on his part – patients who are asleep are unlikely to be critically ill. Her temperature at 9 p.m. had been normal, at 37°C.

At 4.15 a.m. Savita, and Praveen, who was spending the night on a mattress beside his wife, were awake and Savita was feeling 'cold and shivery'. Her temperature was noted as 37.7°C, slightly elevated, and she was given 1 gramme of paracetamol with water to bring it down. Pulse and blood pressure were not recorded at this time. It was not documented at the time, but in her later statement the midwife recalled that Savita was 'shivering and her teeth were chattering'. At 4.20 a.m. Savita vomited, and she and Praveen were given extra blankets, because the room was noted to be cold. The paracetamol appeared to be working: at 5.00 a.m. her temperature was 37.5°C on recheck. The midwife recorded that she 'appeared comfortable and expressed no further complaints'.

However, her shivering and chattering teeth were likely signs of a rigor (feeling of chill despite fever) and indicative of a serious developing infection. Many of us will be familiar with this sensation with onset of flu, for example. It was, however, an error on the part of the nurse not to check Savita's pulse and blood pressure at 4.20 a.m. and call a doctor to see her.

At 6.30 a.m. on the morning of Wednesday, 24 October, Savita's chart shows that she was critically ill. Her temperature had risen to 39.6°C, her heart-rate was 160, and her blood pressure was 94/55. She was feeling weak and had 'general body aches'.

The SHO who had been called at 1.00 a.m. was on the ward with another sick patient and went immediately to see her. Oxygen was administered, cold compresses were applied, and a cannula was inserted. On examination she was tender in the lower abdomen. A foul-smelling discharge was observed that gave immediate cause for concern. The doctor noted his clinical impression as '?chorioamnio-nitis and rule out ?sepsis'.* Chorioamnionitis is an infection of the lining of the womb and the membranes surrounding the baby.

The doctor phoned the registrar to discuss the case, but she was occupied on the delivery suite at the time and could not attend. Savita was commenced on the internationally recommended antibiotic regime and blood tests were taken. At 7.00 a.m. she was noted to be feeling 'slightly better', and her temperature was now 37.9°C. An ECG was performed.

By the time the consultant saw her on the ward round at 8.25 a.m., Savita's condition had only marginally improved. Her temperature was 37.9°C, her pulse rate was 144, and at 100/55 her blood pressure was normal for a pregnant woman. The presumed diagnosis was chorioamnionitis and another antibiotic was added. A white blood cell count was normal.

The consultant discussed a termination of pregnancy with Savita and Praveen: if her condition did not improve, it would have to be considered; however, at this point, it was documented, a fetal heart-beat was still present.

I observed in my report that '[I]t was clear that Mrs Halappanavar developed clinical signs of chorioamnionitis and SIRS (System Inflammatory Response Syndrome).' SIRS is the first stage of sepsis. The most recent RCOG guidelines on 'Bacterial Sepsis in Pregnancy', issued in April 2012, recommended that five steps should be taken within six hours of identification of sepsis.

1. *Blood cultures should be obtained prior to antibiotic administration.* This was done. (These subsequently grew ESBL-*E. coli*. It takes a few days to grow and identify an organism causing an infection. While waiting for lab results, the treating doctors proceeded to Step 2 here.)

2. *A broad-spectrum antibiotic should be administered within one hour.* This was done with the administration of co-amoxiclav at 7.30 a.m. and metronidazole at 8.30 a.m. Dr Susan Knowles, a consultant microbiologist at Holles Street, however, had given evidence the previous week that, although consistent

---

* Use of a question mark is standard medical notation preceding a firm diagnosis.

with the UK's 'Surviving Sepsis Guidelines', this combination was not strong enough to cover the likely infecting organisms. (The antibiotic administered by the Galway team was accepted internationally for use in such situations.* When Savita's infection did not respond to it, her doctors added another one to what she was getting already, but it, too, proved ineffectual.)

3. *Serum lactate should be measured.* This was done and the level was elevated.

4. *In the event of low blood pressure and/or a serum lactate greater than 4* [it was 8.8], *additional fluids (crystalloid) should be administered. If the low blood pressure does not respond, then additional medication should be administered.* This was done, and when Savita's blood pressure fell to 76/46 at 12.00 p.m. the intravenous fluid flow was increased.

5. *In the event of persistent low blood pressure, despite fluid resuscitation and/or lactate greater than 4, those caring for the patient should achieve specific targets for the patient's central venous pressure and central or mixed venous oxygen saturation.* This would require transfer to an intensive care unit.

A full blood count from the test taken at 6.30 a.m. showed a dramatically low white cell count of 1.7, indicating that Savita was heading for septic shock, a condition carrying a 60 per cent mortality rate.

In my opinion, the needle on the dial was over on the far right from 6.30 a.m. onwards on the Wednesday morning. From that point there was, demonstrably, a developing real and substantial risk to Savita's life. As I said in my evidence, '[T]his was clearly recognized by Dr Astbury, who discussed with Mrs Halappanavar and her husband the possibility of the need to terminate the pregnancy.'

In the case of a pregnancy and the development of severe sepsis, emptying the uterus is part of the treatment. Sadly, the locus of the sepsis is the contents of the womb, i.e., the baby the patient is miscarrying. Once delivery occurs the patient's condition usually improves dramatically, since the source of the infection has been removed.

---

* Cases like that of Savita can draw attention to ineffectual treatment regimes and result in review and change.

However, the decision at the ward round was to wait for the results of the blood tests and to see if Savita's condition would continue to improve, since there had been a slight improvement since 6.30 a.m. The fetal heartbeat was still present and this influenced the decision-making process.

By the time I gave my evidence I had read the transcripts of each day of the inquest up to that point. On Day Two, Dr Astbury had been crystal clear in her evidence as to how the law had influenced her judgement. When Praveen's senior counsel, Eugene Gleeson, put it to her that, although another doctor had told Savita that miscarriage was inevitable, she was still holding out for fetal viability, she replied: 'I am waiting because the law states that in the absence of risk to the life of the mother there is no reason to intervene.'

She was then asked if she felt in any way 'constrained or inhibited by Irish law in terms of the treatment [she] could afford Savita'.

She replied, 'Yes. Because termination of pregnancy, which is what she was requesting, is not legal in the context in which she requested it.'

Gleeson next asked if it could be inferred from her response 'that if these events had happened in a neighbouring country such as England that Savita would have had her termination on the Monday or perhaps on the Tuesday, upon request'.

'Yes,' said Dr Astbury. 'Patients are usually offered, as I understand it, if it's under twenty weeks termination is permitted, patients are offered either the option of termination or continuing with the pregnancy.'

'So just by a geographical mischance Savita found herself in this dreadful situation?' Gleeson asked.

'Well, that is the law in this country,' Dr Astbury replied. 'The law in Ireland does not permit termination even if there is no prospect of viability.'

Dr Astbury was correct in her interpretation, and her testimony laid bare just how Irish law on abortion worked in practice.

During the Wednesday morning Savita was nursed in a single room by one midwife who kept the door closed. Savita became progressively sicker as the morning progressed, but the midwife did not alert anyone to her deteriorating condition. At 1 p.m. she was relieved by a student midwife for a lunch break. This student midwife took the immediate action that should have been taken several hours earlier by her colleague. The student found that Savita's blood pressure had fallen from 100/55 at 8.50 a.m. to 73/38 at 1 p.m. Savita was moved to a single room closer to the nurse's station so that she could be kept under closer observation. The consultant was called and came immediately. She found Savita's blood pressure to have fallen further, to 60/30, pulse was 150, and temperature was 37.3°C, and she was also having difficulty breathing.

As I commented in my report to the inquest: '[D]ue to the legal situation regarding termination of pregnancy in Ireland Dr Astbury felt it necessary to obtain a second opinion and signature on the chart from the clinical director (CD) in the event the fetal heartbeat was present prior to proceeding with termination of pregnancy.' The CD agreed that at this stage termination was medically necessary, and asked whether the consultant wanted her to write a note in the chart supporting this decision.

Before proceeding with either a termination or a note in the chart, they decided to check if the fetal heartbeat was still present. A scan shortly before 2 p.m. confirmed that the fetal heart had stopped. The baby was now dead. At this time Savita was in septic shock and the priority was to stabilize her and then deliver the baby.

A microbiologist recommended the addition of further antibiotics. An anaesthetist was consulted, as it was clear that Savita needed to be transferred to the critical care unit (CCU). However, there was no room at this time in the CCU, so she was transferred initially to the gynaecology operating theatre and then at 3.15 p.m. to the high dependency unit. During the course of inserting intravenous lines she miscarried at 4.20 p.m.

My report concluded after Savita delivered her dead baby, as her further care was not my area of expertise.

Twelve hours after miscarrying, Savita was transferred to the intensive care unit, at approximately 3 a.m. on Thursday, 25 October. Despite the full panoply of intensive care, she died at 12.45 a.m. on Sunday, 28 October. The cause of death was multi-organ failure as a result of septic shock due to a septic miscarriage.

My conclusion was that, had Savita's pregnancy been terminated on Monday, 22 October, or Tuesday, 23 October, it is highly likely, on the balance of probabilities, that she would not have died. From the early hours of 24 October Savita had developed sepsis, severe sepsis and septic shock in rapid sequence. The delay in terminating as a consequence of the law allowed the sepsis to take hold, and the sepsis killed her.

Tragically, the locus of the sepsis in Savita's body was in her womb. Had she been delivered, the source of the infection would have been removed. However, termination of pregnancy before the sepsis took hold was not a practical proposition because of the law.

There were a number of deficiencies in care to which I devoted a very large part of my report, specifically the failure to take and record her vital signs consistently, failure to follow up the elevated white blood cell count found on the Sunday, poor note-keeping, and the still unexplained delay in alerting medical staff to the precipitous drop in her blood pressure on the Wednesday morning. None of these on their own was likely to have resulted in Savita's death. Cumulatively, however, they resulted in a delay in appropriate treatment of several hours, and it is well known that each hour in delay in appropriate treatment for sepsis increases the mortality rate by 6 per cent.

Nevertheless, I concluded, based on all the evidence, that there was a strong argument that even if appropriate intervention had commenced in the early hours of 24 October, the outcome would not have been any different. The problem for Savita was that she had a very aggressive organism that resulted in a severe and rapid onset of septic shock. Once the body goes into septic shock, it is extremely difficult to deal with. It can cause multi-organ failure, as it did with Savita. Despite all best efforts by the UHG intensive care team, her life could not be saved.

'The real problem,' I told the inquest, 'was the inability to terminate the pregnancy prior to Savita developing a real and substantial risk of death. By that time it was, effectively, too late to save her life.'

8.   The Eighth Amendment in the spotlight

I had thought long and hard about the words I used in my conclusion to Savita's inquest. I was fairly certain that effectively attributing her death to the Eighth Amendment would provoke a reaction. From the witness box I could see journalists rush out of the room, presumably to file reports, while others typed rapidly on their laptops. Jane was sitting at the back of the courtroom and told me that a group of women who had come in after lunch 'dressed for a wedding or the races' had been steadily barracking me for the previous few minutes. She would later recognize two of them as anti-abortion campaigners.

Predictably, the anti-abortion lobby responded with fury to my conclusion. The medical director of the Pro Life Campaign, Dr Berry Kiely, told the *Irish Times* the next day that 'the manner in which those seeking the introduction of abortion legislation based on the X case ruling have exploited the tragic death of Savita Halappanavar all along . . . [is] . . . little short of shameless.'

The anti-abortion lobby group the Life Institute published a blog on their website within hours titled 'Who is Peter Boylan?' It attacked my professional integrity and claimed that my views were not supported by 'top doctors', and that I did not represent a body of doctors in making my claim. Campaigners told Kitty Holland when she was researching her book on the case that they were frustrated that the 'Boylan narrative' dominated the coverage of the inquest. (This tactic of attempting to isolate me would continue over the coming years. I would be portrayed as the outlier. Some of my more elderly medical colleagues may even have believed this.)

On Friday, 19 April, the jury delivered a unanimous verdict of death due to medical misadventure. The jury strongly endorsed the nine recommendations of the coroner, Ciaran McLoughlin, including a suggestion that the Irish Medical Council lay out exactly when a doctor can intervene to save the life of a mother in similar circumstances. The coroner had earlier said that he was prohibited from making recommendations about changing the law, but in his findings he went as far as he could in referring to the criminal sanction that could be levied on a doctor for breaking the law, as well as erasure from the Medical Register, commenting that 'Doctors who practise medicine with the utmost good faith and to the highest professional standards and in the service of patients should not have to labour under the threat of these sanctions.' I read this as a rebuke to the legislative vacuum of the previous two decades.

Dr Kiely of the Pro Life Campaign, completely ignoring Dr Astbury's evidence, responded by blaming 'system failures and communications shortcomings [which] delayed the moment at which the medical team recognized the seriousness of Savita's condition'.

An RTÉ *Prime Time* programme on the inquest saw me in debate with Professor John Bonnar of Trinity College. John was one of the architects of the Eighth Amendment and, despite our philosophical differences, we had a good professional and personal relationship. His line was that he would have had no difficulty personally with terminating the pregnancy once Savita was ill. But that was precisely the problem with Irish law: we had to wait until the mother was so ill that her life was in danger, and the only way of averting that danger was to terminate the pregnancy, before we could lawfully terminate the pregnancy. It was a uniquely Irish Catch-22.

On Marian Finucane's RTÉ Sunday morning radio programme a couple of days later, I debated with Breda O'Brien, a secondary school teacher and member of the conservative Catholic think tank the Iona Institute. Citing John Bonnar and then falling back on unnamed obstetricians, she claimed that an elevated white cell count on its own justified a termination of pregnancy. This was so ridiculous that when I challenged her, she became flustered and speechless, and Marian Finucane hurriedly moved on.

On 1 May 2013 a group of eleven doctors wrote to the national newspapers, saying that 'much of the public attention appears to have been directed at the expert opinion of Dr Peter Boylan, who suggested that Irish law prevented necessary treatment to save Ms Halappanavar's life. We would suggest that this is a personal view, not an expert one.' It was signed by eight consultant obstetricians, a consultant in emergency medicine, a consultant microbiologist and a consultant anaesthetist. All were known for their anti-abortion views, and some had spoken at anti-abortion events or in the media, including the lead signatory, Dr John Monaghan, as well as Professor Eamon O'Dwyer, Professor John Bonnar and Dr Trevor Hayes.

A key sentence in the letter that continued the discredited line of the white cell count was: 'What we can say with certainty is that where ruptured membranes are accompanied by any clinical or biochemical marker of infection, Irish obstetricians understand they can intervene with early delivery of the baby if necessary.'

Again, this of course was nonsense, and in my reply the next day I drew attention to this: 'This is a truly astonishing statement. It implies that an elevated white blood cell count, which is a non-specific marker of inflammation, on its own would justify a termination of pregnancy. Such an opinion would, not surprisingly, be welcomed by those advocating a complete liberalization of the abortion law in Ireland because, if adopted, would truly "open the floodgates".' They must have known they were talking rubbish, given that the common cold, for example, raises a white blood cell count.

What I found interesting was that the letter had been widely distributed the night before to the general media nationally and internationally and on various social media platforms by John McGuirk, a well-known representative of the Pro Life Campaign. To me this suggested a concerted campaign issuing from No. 6 Gardiner Place in Dublin – the home of the Life Institute and of Youth Defence, among others. It was not an independent initiative by medical professionals.

I subsequently reported all eleven signatories to the Medical Council on the grounds that the letter and its distribution by a known Pro Life campaigner was a concerted and coordinated attack on my professional reputation. I cited three articles of the Medical Council's Guide to Professional Conduct and Ethics for Registered Medical Practitioners: that the letter represented an attempt to 'denigrate' me and was an attempt to 'deliberately damage my practice' and in my opinion represented 'conduct which doctors of experience, competence, and good repute would consider disgraceful and falls short, by commission of the standard of conduct expected among doctors'.

In the course of their responses to the Medical Council none of the signatories admitted knowing John McGuirk. This puzzled me. If none of the signatories knew of McGuirk, how had he managed to get a copy of the letter before publication? Divine intervention perhaps? The Medical Council did not find the doctors guilty of professional misconduct, and I decided not to take the case any further: as far as I was concerned my point had been made.

I had learned something about anti-abortion campaigners, however, that proved useful in the years ahead. They agree a party line on an issue, and then various spokespeople advance it across multiple platforms – radio, television, print and social media – over a few days. When their line is on medical grounds, it is generally unsound and easily refutable, and I took action to counter these moves robustly early. Often I would find that planned interviews were cancelled as the issue ran out of steam once I had given an interview or spoken to producers and journalists.

After the Galway inquest there were three further investigations into Savita's death, one each commissioned by the HSE and the Health Information and Quality Authority (HIQA) respectively, and a 2018 disciplinary hearing into the midwives at UHG by the Nursing and Midwifery Board of Ireland (NMBI). A complaint to the Medical Council in 2015 against Dr Katherine Astbury did not progress beyond a preliminary hearing.

The HSE commissioned an inquiry chaired by Professor Sir Sabaratnam Arulkumaran, then professor and head of obstetrics and gynaecology at St George's, University of London, president of the British Medical Association and former president of both the British and international ob-gyn bodies, RCOG and FIGO.* To his friends and colleagues he is known simply as Arul and is hugely respected. I have known him for many years. (Indeed, in the 1990s he had invited me to be a visiting professor when he was head of department at the National University of Singapore. At the time I was master of the NMH and it wasn't a practical proposition.)

The HSE report was issued on 13 June 2013. At the press conference Arul said that had Savita been in his care in England, she would have been given the option of a termination on her second visit to UHG on Sunday, 21 October, given the impending miscarriage. She would have been advised to terminate her pregnancy once her waters broke at half past midnight on the Monday night into early Tuesday morning due to the risk of infection. As she was in Ireland, where the

---

* The International Federation of Gynecology and Obstetrics.

law prohibited these courses of action, he went on to say that she should have been monitored closely given the risk of sepsis.

'We established that the patient was monitored less frequently than required, that guidelines for the prompt and effective management of sepsis were not adhered to. We also believe that legislative factors affected medical consideration in this case, and that this resulted in a failure to offer all management options to the patient.'

The report expanded on these points over 108 pages. It enumerated failures of clinical management similar to those described in my report to the inquest. It laid out the confusion caused by lack of clarity in Irish law and guidelines, and showed how this had impinged on the doctors' decision-making. The report recommended a series of improvements in clinical guidelines and, crucially, made it clear that, in order to improve the guidelines, there might be a requirement for legal change.

There are no accepted clear local, national or international guidelines on the management of inevitable early second trimester miscarriage [i.e., less than twenty-four weeks] including the management of miscarriage where there is prolonged rupture of the membranes . . . It is recommended that such guidelines be developed for such patients as a matter of urgency and they should be explicit in the guidance given as to when one should offer termination based on symptoms and signs of infection implying increasing health risk to the mother which may even threaten her life. We recognise that such guidelines must be consistent with applicable law and that the guidance so urged may require legal change.

The investigation team is satisfied that concerns about the law, whether clear or not, impacted on the exercise of clinical professional judgement.

There is an immediate and urgent requirement for a clear statement of the legal context in which clinical professional judgement can be exercised in the best medical welfare interests of patients. We recommend that the clinical professional community, health and social care regulators, and the Oireachtas, consider the law including any necessary constitutional change and related administrative, legal and clinical guidelines in relation to the management of inevitable miscarriage in the early second trimester of a pregnancy . . .

I particularly welcomed the recommendation that the Oireachtas address legislative change, as it was what I was advocating.

Needless to say, anti-abortion campaigners focused entirely on the deficiencies in care that Arul and I had detailed, and completely

ignored our conclusion on the impact of the law on Savita's management. We have watched over the years as they have wrongly tried to
claim that Arul's report contradicted mine. In general, this is an
opinion held only among the most extreme anti-choice campaigners
and on the wilder shores of social media.

A further inquiry was conducted by HIQA, which conducted an
'Investigation into the safety, quality and standards of services provided by the Health Service Executive (HSE) to patients, including
pregnant women, at risk of clinical deterioration, including those
provided in University Hospital Galway (UHG) and as reflected in
the care and treatment provided to Savita Halappanavar'.

The HIQA report was published in October 2013. It was critical of
a number of areas of clinical practice as previously outlined in the
inquest and in the HSE report. It also criticized governance arrangements at UHG.

In particular, the HIQA report drew attention to the low numbers
of consultant obstetricians in Ireland by international standards. On
RTÉ's *Morning Ireland* I described this as 'an appalling indictment of
state failure' in relation to the funding of maternity services.

For perhaps the first time in public, the HIQA report referred to
the workload of the midwives on St Monica's Ward during Savita's
admission. It found that the case mix of patients and their care needs
was 'significantly diverse and complex' but said that there was no evidence that hospital management took account of this.

The HIQA report recommended a National Maternity Strategy,
and this was subsequently launched in January 2016. The impact of
the law was excluded from the terms of reference, so there was no
comment on this aspect. This did not stop anti-abortion campaigners
later disingenuously claiming that the report found no legal difficulties with Savita's management.

In 2018 the NMBI initiated a fitness to practise inquiry into the performance of the three midwives who had nursed Savita. The solicitors
acting for the women asked me to give an expert opinion as an obstetrician for the two nurses on-duty overnight during Savita's
admission, and the nurse who was with her during the Wednesday
morning when, inexplicably, medical staff were not alerted to her
deteriorating condition. That nurse was unable to give evidence at

the inquest because of illness and was also unable to provide a statement to the fitness to practise inquiry.

I had been told before the inquest that at least one patient had died on the ward the night Savita became critically ill, and I was aware that the staff had been badly stretched. However, it was only when I was asked to give an expert opinion to the NMBI inquiry that I became fully aware of the truly appalling conditions in which the midwives in Galway were working in autumn 2012.

For the first three nights following Savita's admission, those two midwives alone, one of whom was far advanced herself in pregnancy, were allocated to look after all of the patients on St Monica's. The ward had fifteen inpatient beds, four trolley spaces allocated for day cases, and a clinical examination room that contained an ultrasound scan machine. It was primarily a gynaecology ward, but it could also accommodate antenatal patients in early pregnancy up to twenty weeks gestation including those miscarrying, those with threatened miscarriage, missed miscarriage, inevitable miscarriage and ectopic pregnancies being treated either actively or conservatively. The ward also accommodated pre-operative and post-operative gynaecology patients, including those who had had surgery for cancer.

In addition, all patients presenting with a gynaecology or obstetrics emergency outside the hours of 9.00 a.m. to 5 p.m., Monday to Friday or on Bank Holidays, were directed to St Monica's Ward for assessment.

A month before Savita died, the midwives on St Monica's had collectively expressed their concerns regarding clinical risks in their working environment. On their behalf, the Irish Nurses and Midwives Organisation (INMO) wrote to the assistant director of nursing and midwifery at UHG on 28 September, stating: 'the concern of staff on St Monica's Ward was that staff were overburdened and that this posed a significant potential risk to patients' safety.'

When, for the hearing, I received the details of the patients that two midwives were expected to care for overnight, I was horrified. The nursing care that Savita received during the three nights she was on St Monica's Ward has to be seen and judged in the context of the workload of the medical staff (two junior doctors – a registrar and a senior house officer – were on-duty to deal with problems on the labour ward, perform Caesarean sections and manage whatever came up on the other wards) and the almost impossible standards to which the midwives were expected to adhere.

On the night of Sunday, 21 October, into the morning of Monday, 22 October 2012 – the night Savita was admitted – the ward was extremely busy. There was a very sick patient who had come from the high dependency unit in the General Hospital who needed hourly observation as well as blood transfusions.

There were two terminally ill cancer patients undergoing palliative care. One was agitated all night and trying to get out of bed. A second was on intravenous fluids, intravenous antibiotics and a subcutaneous morphine pump and required full nursing care. She died on the Tuesday morning.

There were five patients recovering from hysterectomies and/or removal of their ovaries, all of which were either abdominal or vaginal. One of these had undergone extensive cancer surgery and been transferred to St Monica's from the high dependency unit. She still required one-to-one care.

A further patient had been readmitted a month after a pelvic-floor repair with abdominal pain and swelling, and was being investigated for ovarian cancer. Yet another patient was recuperating from having an ovarian cyst removed. She was non-compliant with her diabetes, and kept leaving the ward to smoke against advice. She had a psychiatric history, was on a lot of medication, and was confrontational and difficult to manage.

On the obstetric side, there were four patients in addition to Savita. Two women at eleven weeks gestation with vomiting and nausea were receiving intravenous fluids. There was a woman at five weeks gestation with abdominal pain and bleeding, and another, following embryo implantation, who was admitted with abdominal pain.

Patients were not formally allocated to individual midwives on-duty; therefore, if a patient rang the call-bell, whichever midwife was the first to become available was the one who answered. The midwives worked twelve-hour shifts, 8 p.m. to 8 a.m. Due to the high level of activity on the ward that night, they were unable to take an extended meal break.

This was an extraordinary caseload for two midwives to cope with for a continuous twelve-hour period but, unfortunately, all too common in our hospitals.

The same two midwives were on-duty the next night, Monday, 22 October, into Tuesday, 23 October. The ward diary entry noted that a healthcare assistant had come in for one hour early in the night to sit with an agitated patient and another one came at 5.45 a.m. to help reposition a patient, but that was all the help the two midwives got during those twelve hours. The midwives made a note that they felt that there were inadequate staffing levels overnight and that these levels were 'compromising patient care. Night sister aware.'

There were six more patients in addition to those of the previous night. A seventy-year-old patient with a history of ovarian cancer undergoing palliative care had to be nursed in an isolation room because of MRSA.

One woman had undergone a radical hysterectomy during the day for cervical cancer. Another patient had been readmitted with post-operative complications. A woman who was eleven weeks pregnant had abdominal pain due to a degenerating fibroid in her uterus. This patient required regular pethidine and other nursing care.

Another patient was at sixteen weeks gestation with a threatened miscarriage, bleeding and lower abdominal pain. At the inquiry the midwife reported that this woman was 'highly intoxicated and needed close nursing observation'. She was residing in a Simon Community facility, and through the night there were 'lengthy discussions with the Simon Community about this patient'.

Things weren't looking any more promising on St Monica's for the next night – Tuesday, 23 October, into Wednesday, 24 October. The following email was sent by a nursing manager to the assistant director of nursing at 6.44 p.m.

Subject Re: Sick Leave

Dear A,

Just to let you know that B was sick today on a long day and C on a late shift. It is extremely short staffed, I do not know when B or C will be back D has sent in a sick cert for the rest of the week and up to 29th October 2012 inclusive. I rang the office but there was no one. A student midwife came from the labour ward to help for a few hours, one of the direct entry students E was unable to come on-duty due to her not feeling well today. A patient passed away at 08.40 and a lot of time was spent dealing with the family etc. I asked F to stay on but she could not, due to other commitments. I stayed on myself as there was no other option. I want to mention also that G [one of the midwives on-duty in St Monica's on the relevant nights] who is now fairly advanced in her pregnancy and H [the other midwife on-duty in St Monica's during the relevant period] put through a difficult night last night. I had asked for a care assistant earlier in the day to assist them as I knew that she would be needed. Unfortunately a person only came for a short while, the staff in the morning were very upset that they got no one. The patient in Room 8 took up a nurse on her own as she was extremely ill, as I stated she died that morning. Also there was another patient very ill that night started on TPN today. I have asked nursing support to send the night staff someone tonight.

Regards
K.

When the two night-duty midwives – the same two who had worked the previous two nights – went back on-duty for their twelve-hour shift just over an hour later, at 8 p.m., they both broke down and cried when they realized they were on their own again with little prospect of additional nursing support. As it transpired, no nursing support was provided overnight when Savita became critically ill in the early hours of Wednesday morning. And in the meantime, a further patient who had a miscarriage treated surgically late on Tuesday evening returned to St Monica's at 11.50 p.m. and required nursing care overnight.

The INMO code of practice states that: 'The aim of the nursing profession is to give the highest standard of care possible to patients. Any circumstances which could place patients/clients in jeopardy or which militate against safe standards of practice should be made known to appropriate persons or authorities.'

The midwives had expressed their concerns to the hospital management on several occasions, including at a nursing meeting on 28 September. This was clearly a long-standing problem.

The INMO code further states that: 'The nurse shares the responsibility of care with colleagues and must have regard to the workload of, and the pressure on, professional colleagues and subordinates and take appropriate action if these are seen to be such as to constitute abuse of the individual practitioner and/or to jeopardize safe standards of practice.'

In my view, asking two nurses to care for so many sick patients over a twelve-hour period could very reasonably be regarded as constituting an abuse of the individual practitioner. The staff levels on the nights in question were inadequate for the caseload of patients.

Given that so many on the anti-abortion side of the argument relied on the shortcomings in Savita's care to say that her death had nothing to do with the Eighth Amendment, it is worth considering what might have happened if the midwife on-duty had taken Savita's vital signs at 4.15 a.m. on Wednesday morning and found her pulse to be significantly elevated. The failure to do this was identified as a deficiency in care by me at the inquest, and also in the HSE and HIQA inquiries.

It is likely that she would have called the doctor on-duty, who would have reviewed Savita as soon as he could and probably commenced the antibiotic regime at 4.30 a.m. rather than at 6.30 a.m. As it transpired, however, the medications that were prescribed were ineffective for the particular infection that developed, despite being the internationally accepted regime. Thus it is hard to see how there would have been a change in the eventual outcome.

Another deficiency identified was the failure to check vital signs (pulse, temperature, blood pressure and oxygen saturation level) every four hours. The check due at 2.00 a.m. on the Tuesday morning was not done. However, given that there was no significant change in the vital signs between 9.40 p.m. on Monday and 6 a.m. on Tuesday, it is reasonable to conclude, on the balance of probabilities, that Savita's vital signs would not have been worse at 2.00 a.m.

The failure to make recordings at 2.00 a.m. has to be seen in the context of the workload. Given the extreme pressure, it was incumbent on the midwives to prioritize care for patients, with those in greatest need being of highest priority. On the night in question, Monday into Tuesday, it is clear that Savita was not critically ill; and it is also clear from the list of other patients whom the midwives were caring for that some of these were critically ill, and indeed one died on the morning of 23 October.

In my opinion to the NMBI's fitness to practise inquiry I stated that the midwives did the best they could in extremely difficult circumstances. Responsibility for providing adequate staffing levels does not rest with the midwives on-duty and, in my view, they should not be held personally responsible for the shortfall in nursing care that Savita experienced. The midwives were not found guilty of professional misconduct.

The Medical Council held a preliminary inquiry into the conduct of Dr Katherine Astbury following a complaint in 2013 from Councillor Pádraig Conneely of Galway. During these proceedings the committee considered an independent expert report of December 2014 from Dr Jane Norman, professor of maternal and fetal health at the University of Edinburgh. Dr Norman concluded: 'Katherine Astbury's management of Savita Halappanavar was appropriate; in terms of clinical decision-making and treatment options . . . She involved colleagues from other specialities appropriately . . . I do not think the actions of Dr Katherine Astbury fulfil the criteria for poor professional performance or professional misconduct.' The Medical Council concluded in March 2015 that they would take no further action.

At the end of all five investigations, there could be little doubt that had Savita Halappanavar's pregnancy been terminated on either the Monday or the Tuesday, she would not have died. It was also clear that there were serious systemic problems in University Hospital Galway that gave rise to an environment that was not conducive to patient safety. As the HIQA inquiry made clear, these were not confined to Galway. The events in Galway shone a spotlight on chronic underinvestment in Irish maternity services over decades.

So, is it possible to determine who or what was responsible for Savita's death?

Was it the nursing staff who were asked to do the virtually impossible by monitoring the number of sick patients on St Monica's over those three days and nights?

Was it the nursing management who failed, or were unable, to provide sufficient staff?

Was it hospital management who failed to employ sufficient nursing staff?

Was the Saolta Group★ at fault for not ensuring better clinical and corporate governance in the hospital?

Was it the state that failed to make the necessary investment in nursing numbers?

Was it the junior doctor who failed to make sure the white blood cell count taken on the day of admission was followed up?

Was it the junior doctor who failed to attend Savita earlier on the night of the 23rd when requested by the nursing staff? Should they have ignored the other patients they were attending to go to check Savita?

Should the nurse have asked the consultant on call to go and see Savita if the junior doctor wasn't able to because of pressure of work?

Was the hospital management at fault, because it was their responsibility to ensure that there were sufficient junior staff on call at all times?

Was the junior doctor at fault for not waking Savita at 1 a.m. to check vital signs?

Should the consultant not have been better able to interpret the Supreme Court ruling on the X case?

Was the RCOG at fault for not having more appropriate management guidelines in cases such as Savita's, particularly in relation to antibiotic treatment?

Was the state responsible because legislation had not been enacted to clarify for doctors when it was legal to terminate a pregnancy without fear of a jail sentence?

When things go wrong, it is a natural human tendency to seek to blame somebody, almost always, however, there is usually no one person totally responsible for a bad outcome. It is almost always a series of minor errors combined that is the cause. If we are to learn from bad outcomes, it is important to try to discover why these errors occurred.

As I pointed out in my evidence to the inquest, there were deficiencies in Savita's care – undoubtedly what happened to her reflected the effects of decades of underfunding in our maternity and gynaecology

★ The hospital group for the west and north-west of Ireland.

services. But above that her death shone a light on the malign influence of the Eighth Amendment. Had it been possible to accede to Savita's wish to terminate her pregnancy when she knew that she was losing her baby, there is no doubt that she would not have died, and the question of deficiencies would never have arisen. Ultimately, the presence of the Eighth Amendment cost Savita her life.

9. The government under pressure

At the time of Savita Halappanavar's inquest in April 2013, I was a little over three years away from retirement and increasingly determined to do everything I could to help eradicate the Eighth Amendment from our Constitution. It had poisoned the practice of obstetrics in Ireland and was harming women. Irish women were not equal citizens of their own country while the shadow of the Eighth fell over them. In the wake of Savita's tragic death, the amendment was now in the spotlight and unlikely to fade into the background again.

The previous year, as I have written earlier, well before Savita's death, the Minister for Health, Dr James Reilly, had asked me to sit on an expert group asked to give the government options so it could comply with a landmark European Court of Human Rights ruling against the state in the matter of abortion.

The case went back to August 2005, when three women living in Ireland lodged a complaint to the ECHR alleging that restrictions on abortion in Ireland were in breach of their human rights under a number of articles of the European Convention on Human Rights. All of the applicants were women who unintentionally became pregnant and who travelled to the UK for abortions.

The first applicant, A, was a woman living in poverty and the mother of four children who were in care. When she became pregnant again, she was attempting to reunite her family and felt unable to cope with a fifth child.

The second applicant, B, was a single woman who became pregnant when emergency contraception failed and who believed that she could not care for a child at that time in her life.

The third applicant, C, had been treated for cancer for three years. When she became unintentionally pregnant, she was in remission but was unable to obtain clear medical advice as to the effect of the pregnancy on her health or life, or the effect of the medical treatment on the fetus. She was also afraid that the pregnancy might lead to a recurrence of the cancer and so she decided to have an abortion.

In its judgment of 16 December 2010, the ECHR did not find a right to abortion within the convention. Therefore the women's case rested on how existing Irish law affected them. The court refused A's and B's applications, finding that they had sought abortions for reasons of health and/or well-being (i.e., their lives were not at risk so the X case ruling did not apply). However, the court held that there had been a violation in respect of C, because she could not get clear information about her rights in a situation where she believed there was a risk to her life if her pregnancy continued. It was, the court ruled, a violation of her right to privacy. Miss C was awarded damages of €15,000 for the 'considerable suffering and anxiety' caused to her by the legal uncertainty.

This finding put the Irish government under pressure once more. It had to clarify the circumstances in which a pregnancy could be terminated to save a woman's life. As part of the judgment Ireland was required to establish an expert group to address the issue with a view to making recommendations to government.

Thus, at the beginning of 2012, twenty-nine years after the insertion of the Eighth Amendment into the Constitution, and after a legislative vacuum of twenty years since the X case, the ECHR had forced the Irish government to take its first very limited step to address the confusion about abortion law in Ireland.

The expert group was chaired by Mr Justice Sean Ryan and had representatives from obstetrics, psychiatry, general practice, law, policy, and professional standards for doctors and midwives. We met nine times from January to October 2012.

Our terms of reference were solely to look at the implications of the ECHR judgment with regard to Miss C. We were not asked to consider abortion for any reason other than as a threat to the woman's life that could be averted only by termination of pregnancy. Some thought that this was regrettable but in my opinion it was better to move incrementally. I felt that the introduction of legislation that made termination legal in certain very restricted circumstances would help to change the atmosphere in Ireland with regard to provision of the service. The sky would not fall in and the proverbial floodgates, which are much feared by Irish conservatives, would once again fail to open.

The report of the expert group was delivered to government on the evening of Tuesday, 13 November 2012. It presented four options: the non-statutory option of guidelines only; and three statutory options – regulations alone, legislation alone or legislation combined with regulation. Given the mood of public anger and shock that followed the news that broke about Savita Halappanavar's death the following day, the government came under severe pressure to finally legislate for the X case. It appeared to me that, while the death of Savita had been a huge tragedy, it provided the government, particularly the more conservative Fine Gael partner, with political 'cover' to proceed with legislation on the foot of our report. Given politicians' propensity for commissioning expert reports and then disregarding their findings, it's likely this might have happened again had Savita's death not caused an outcry.

A month later, on 18 December 2012, when the Cabinet decided that its preferred option to give effect to the X case judgment was a combination of legislation and regulation, the issue of suicide immediately raised political difficulties. Around twenty Fine Gael TDs indicated that they would not support the inclusion in any legislation of the threat of suicide as a basis for abortion. The Minister for Health, however, maintained that legislation would have to cover suicide, since the Supreme Court had been very clear on the issue.

The Oireachtas Joint Committee on Health and Children arranged hearings for 9, 10 and 11 January 2013 to hear respectively from doctors, lawyers, and representatives from religious and non-religious organizations.

The Catholic Church and the anti-abortion lobby were galvanized. The day before the start of the hearings Pope Benedict XVI expressed 'dismay' at the proposed introduction of abortion legislation in 'various countries, even those of Christian tradition', while the bishop of Kilmore, Leo O'Reilly, described the government's proposal to legislate as representing 'the first step on the road to a culture of death'.

On the first day of the hearings, Dr Rhona Mahony, master of Holles Street, made a strong statement calling for doctors to be allowed to make decisions based on medical fact, with legal protection. One particular comment – 'I want to know that I will not go to jail, and I want to know that she [the patient] will not go to jail' – caught public attention. So, too, did her pointed question: 'What is a substantial risk to life during pregnancy – a 10 per cent risk? – an 8 per cent risk? – a 1 per cent risk of dying? The interpretation of risk is not the same for all people.' Meanwhile, the Rotunda's Dr Sam Coulter-Smith said the hospital dealt with about forty cases a year of pregnant women with life-threatening illnesses and five or six cases 'where interruption of the pregnancy is required to save the mother's life'.

The psychiatrist Dr Anthony McCarthy of Holles Street told the Committee that, although suicide in pregnancy is rare, it does happen. He said that, while discussion around, for example, cyberbullying and suicide generated great public sympathy, the pejorative tone of the discussion of pregnant women and suicide was 'horrifying'.

Dr McCarthy made very clear to the Committee the difference between suicidal ideation and suicidal intent. In the first instance a woman has a passive death wish, or ideas about ending her life that may be occasional, frequent or constant. 'Suicidal intent,' he emphasized, 'is different. Here the person has an intention or plan to kill herself. It is no longer just an idea.' It was likely that some women would develop suicidal intent if denied an abortion, but the 'safety valve' of the ease of access to abortion in the UK made this a rare event.

Not all obstetricians were in favour of proceeding with legislation. Dr John Monaghan of Portiuncula Hospital in Ballinasloe, for example, was alarmed by the publicity that followed the appearances of Dr Mahony and Dr Coulter-Smith and drafted a letter to the Committee arguing against the introduction of abortion in Ireland. He circulated it in advance to members of the Institute of Obstetricians and Gynaecologists, asking if any of us would like to be associated with it. I replied, saying that the Oireachtas hearings were an effort by our legislators to understand better how they should frame the legislation that they are committed to enacting. 'I find it difficult,' I wrote, 'to understand objections to the enacting of legislation designed to better protect women's lives. Surely that is at the core of our profession?' I urged Dr Monaghan to reconsider sending his letter.

On Saturday, 19 January 2013, some 25,000 people attended a 'Unite for Life' vigil in Dublin organized by the Pro Life Campaign.

On the political front two senior Fine Gael figures spoke out against any legislation that included suicide as grounds for abortion. Lucinda Creighton, Minister of State for European Affairs, proposed a bill to deal with the issue that excluded suicide. She told RTÉ radio that she wanted to ensure that 'We don't open the floodgates.' In mid February former Taoiseach John Bruton made an intervention that cannot have been welcomed by his successor, Enda Kenny. He declared that it was 'not consistent with the plain words of the Constitution' to include the threat of suicide in the terms of the legislation that would permit abortion where a woman's life was at risk.

On 23 April, five days after the jury returned a unanimous verdict of medical misadventure in Savita's Halappanavar's inquest, the draft legislation of what was then called the Protection of Maternal Life Bill was brought before the Cabinet, and exactly a week later the government published the General Scheme of the Protection of Life During Pregnancy Bill 2013. Oireachtas Committee hearings were scheduled to consider this draft legislation over three days in May.

On the first day of the hearings, Friday, 17 May, a number of doctors representing the various professional bodies, as well as the maternity hospitals, were invited before the Committee. I appeared with Sam Coulter-Smith and Rhona Mahony.

My aim was to turn the spotlight on the hypocritical nature of our Constitution on the question of abortion. I said I thought it was bizarre and contradictory to propose that a woman be sentenced to fourteen years in prison for accepting medical advice in the state and having a termination, particularly so when she had 'the constitutional protection of this country if she goes to the UK and has the same procedure'. It made no sense at all, I told the Committee.

The overall situation placed the woman in question in the highly unsatisfactory position of having doctors who were unsure as to whether or not they would be breaking the law if they felt they had to intervene to save her life. And women had no input into the decision about whether or not they were willing to accept the risk of death or wished to have a termination to avoid that risk.

My thinking was strongly influenced by the experience of reviewing Savita's clinical course for her inquest. Some women would be willing to take any risk to achieve a successful pregnancy, while for others the risk would be too great. I gave the Committee an example of two forty-year-old women with severe diabetes whose pregnancies put them at serious risk of kidney disease and deterioration in their eyesight. One might have had a series of unsuccessful attempts at IVF but have finally achieved an ongoing pregnancy and so might have been willing to accept any risk. The other woman might have had four other young children at home and would not have been willing to accept the risk. Personal circumstances influence one's attitude to risk, but the current situation did not allow for a nuanced approach, and neither did it allow for any input by the woman herself, a unique situation in the practice of obstetrics.

I observed that some campaigners were attempting to suggest that late terminations would be performed in Irish hospitals if the legislation was passed, implying that doctors would deliberately kill an unborn baby capable of existence outside the uterus. Some of the more extreme groups were even suggesting that newborn babies might be killed. These views, I said, were clearly extremist, had no basis in fact and were, quite frankly, insulting.

Dr Mahony told the Committee that in her experience the majority of women did not wish to lose their babies, but nor did they want to die. The bill, she said, was not about suicide in pregnancy, but 'about saving women's lives, regardless of whether the risk to life is physical or mental'.

Dr Coulter-Smith said that the suicide clause raised a number of issues. Relying on evidence from some psychiatrists that there was no data to show that abortion was a treatment for suicide, his comments were picked up as a division between doctors, but in fact he welcomed the rest of the bill. In the next session, however, Dr John Monaghan said that, unlike the previous session's obstetricians, he was not happy to take the expert advice of a psychiatrist on the issue of suicide.

Some anti-abortion members of the Oireachtas continued to drive a narrative that women would manipulate the provision for termination where it was allowed in cases of a risk of suicide and that this would result in a huge increase in terminations. The implication was that women could not be trusted. I found this objectionable.

As the debate continued in Leinster House, the Catholic Church upped the ante. Archbishop Eamon Martin of Armagh told a Sunday newspaper that politicians who knowingly introduced legislation 'aiding and abetting abortion' would be denied communion. The archbishop of Dublin, Diarmuid Martin, once again took a more conciliatory view, saying that he believed communion 'should not . . . be used for publicity reasons by anybody'.

In mid June the government announced that it intended to enact legislation before the summer recess. It published a revised bill that restated the general prohibition on abortion in Ireland, including that it would be an offence to intentionally destroy unborn human life, and with guilty parties – including the woman – liable to a fine or imprisonment for a term not exceeding fourteen years, or both.

However, for the first time, it also set out processes to establish the circumstances in which there was a real and substantial risk to the life of a woman.

In the case of that risk to a woman's life arising from a physical health condition, an obstetrician/gynaecologist and a second relevant specialist would have to jointly agree and certify that the termination of pregnancy was the only treatment that would save her life.

In the case of an immediate risk to the woman's life, one doctor could make the decision.

In the case of a real and substantial risk to a woman's life arising from suicide, three doctors – one obstetrician/gynaecologist and two psychiatrists – would have to jointly and unanimously agree and certify that the termination of pregnancy was the only treatment that would save her life.

Additionally, an appeals process would entitle a woman to a review of a decision when the assessing doctors did not certify that a termination was permissible.

While conscientious objection for individual doctors was quite properly retained, with the requirement to provide for transfer of care in such an instance, an earlier proposal that institutions could opt out was dropped. The list of institutions approved for carrying out terminations was also widened from nineteen to twenty-five, to include major teaching hospitals that did not have maternity units. Minister James Reilly made the point clearly on radio that no medical institution would be allowed to refuse a woman a termination if her life was in danger.

For Pro Life campaigners, however, even this limited legislation was too much, with one Senator – Rónán Mullen – suggesting that the legislation might 'incentivise a medical practitioner to opt for an abortion instead of an early inducement [*sic*] so as to avoid questions of civil liability on foot of the disablement of a child'. Increasingly, the tactics of the Pro Life Campaign became about placing the 'blame' for abortion on doctors, reflecting their refusal to contemplate abortion in any circumstances whatsoever, and possibly as a way of avoiding discussion of the very difficult cases like Savita's. (These comments were a foretaste of the quite reprehensible statements that would issue from the anti-abortion lobby in the years ahead.)

The Protection of Life During Pregnancy Act was approved in the Dáil on 12 July by 127 votes to 31. Six of those who voted against it were pro-choice TDs who thought the legislation did not go far enough. It was then passed unamended in the Seanad by 39 votes to 14, and on 30 July President Michael D. Higgins signed it into law.

A huge amount of effort had gone into the Act (the January Oireachtas hearings alone had produced a 1,000-page report). But now, for the first time, from 1 January 2014, doctors had legislation to guide us as to when it was legal to terminate a pregnancy in Ireland; we would no longer have to interpret the Constitution. And, although the legislation was extremely restrictive, I felt it would help change attitudes towards abortion, both in the general population and among medical staff.

In the first four years following the commencement of the law the numbers of terminations ranged from 26 in 2014 to 15 in 2017 (the last year for which figures are available). The total number performed on the basis of a risk of suicide was 9 in those first four years – confirmation, if confirmation was needed, that neither women nor doctors were abusing the system.

10. An extraordinary transformation in Ireland's abortion debate

Three months after the Protection of Life During Pregnancy Act came into effect a case arose that in its horror demonstrated all too clearly that Ireland's abortion law was still failing women, especially the most vulnerable.

The young woman who became known as Ms Y was a refugee from a particularly violent war zone in Africa. She arrived in Ireland on 28 March 2014. She had been raped repeatedly, and did not know she was pregnant until a test was done as part of a health screening check in early April. A social worker at the refugee reception centre referred her to the Irish Family Planning Association (IFPA). On 8 April she was seen at the IFPA and the pregnancy was again confirmed. Ms Y, who did not speak English, became very distressed, but not (yet) suicidal, and requested a termination. The legal situation in Ireland was explained to her through an interpreter: she was not eligible for a termination in Ireland because her life was not at risk.

An ultrasound scan on 11 April dated the pregnancy at eight weeks and four days. Because of her refugee status, the Immigration Council of Ireland was contacted to explore the logistics of arranging for her to travel outside the state for an abortion. The ICI explained that getting travel documents from the Irish Naturalization and Immigration Service could be a lengthy process.

At the end of May, the question of adoption was discussed at a consultation at the IFPA. She was now fifteen weeks pregnant. Her response was clear – she would 'rather die than have this baby'. Ms Y was given forms to fill out, and it was explained to her that she would need nearly €1,300 in order to travel to the Netherlands for a termination. (The cost would be less in the Netherlands than in the UK.)

The process was becoming positively Kafkaesque. Ms Y spoke no English, had no money, was severely traumatized and was living in direct provision accommodation. To travel she needed a passport (€80), photos signed by a garda, a visa for the country she was to travel to (€60, with both Dutch and English embassies requiring at least ten separate pieces of documentation before a visa could be issued, while, additionally, the British required an email account to receive and send a ten-page application form), hotel (€100), flights (€300) and clinic fee (€700). She would have to arrange the appointment in the clinic herself, since the Regulation of Information Act 1995 specifically prohibited anyone making an appointment on her behalf. She also needed a Garda National Immigration card number, an up-to-date bank account showing sufficient funds to cover her journey, a copy of medical travel insurance, details of booked accommodation and details of return travel arrangements that could be secured only by making a credit card payment. Temporary travel documents from the Irish National Immigration Service also required that she have a PPS number.

Whatever support Ms Y was receiving was from non-governmental organizations – from the moment her pregnancy was confirmed, during the initial health screening, no state agency could offer her any advice or assistance – and because of the law the NGOs could not assist her in organizing a termination. Unable to speak or write English, she could not fill out the documents, and so the travel plans stalled. Around the same time she was reviewed by a doctor and was noted to be very distressed, with 'a strong death-wish'.

In early June Ms Y was seen by a psycho-social worker from the national centre for the rehabilitation of victims of torture in Ireland, Spirasi,★ in order to complete forms required for a medical legal report about her asylum status. On her own initiative she took a ferry to Liverpool around this time in the hope of accessing a termination there. UK immigration officers detained her on arrival and sent her back to Ireland.

In early July, now twenty-one weeks pregnant, she moved to new accommodation, as she did not want people to know about the pregnancy. On a visit to the GP she had been seeing Ms Y said that she wanted to have an abortion and was referred for an outpatient psychiatric assessment. By now she was twenty-two weeks pregnant. The consultant psychiatrist who assessed her explained that it was too late for an abortion. Ms Y responded that she was going to commit suicide and gave details of her plan. The psychiatrist noted the evidence of suicidal intent.

★ Spiritan Asylum Services Initiative.

Ms Y was then transferred to a maternity hospital, where a scan established that she was now twenty-four weeks pregnant. She was made aware that if she tried to leave the hospital, she would be detained under mental health legislation. She went on a hunger strike, and this lasted for five days, until it was agreed that the baby would be delivered in the following days. The psychiatrist who had seen her a week earlier considered that she was at significant risk of suicide, and this was directly related to her unsuccessful efforts to secure an abortion.

The hospital's clinical director and a consultant obstetrician visited Ms Y and explained that the hospital was seeking legal advice, and that this might delay the delivery of her baby. Despite the new legislation the doctors still were uncertain about how to proceed. Their concerns were genuine and justified. The pregnancy was now close to, or at, viability, and they were concerned about the outcome for the baby if delivered so prematurely.

Ms Y refused food and fluids again, and became uncommunicative. Doctors were concerned that she was developing metabolic acidosis, where there is too much acid in body fluids and which can cause coma and death.

In the meantime, the HSE applied to the High Court for permission to forcibly sedate and rehydrate the young woman, and the order was granted. She remained adamant that she would kill herself if the plan to deliver did not proceed. After forty hours with no fluids she saw another psychiatrist who judged her an ongoing suicide risk. Now twenty-six weeks pregnant, she agreed to have a Caesarean section the next day, so the medical staff did not have to proceed with forcible rehydration. More than sixteen weeks had passed since the original pregnancy test and request for termination. With all the various organizations she saw in that time, she was lost to follow-up. No one person or organization could take care of her.

After the Caesarean section, Ms Y's baby was taken to the neonatal care unit. She could not bring herself even to see the child. Seven days later she was discharged from the hospital and returned to her accommodation. The baby was taken into the care of the HSE.

The PLDP Act was supposed to address situations such as this, but the Y case exposed some of the deficiencies in the new legislative environment and made it ever more apparent to me that repeal of the

Eighth was the only rational solution to the recurring dilemmas confronting women, and doctors.

In reflecting on Ms Y's experience, I recalled the report written in 1994 by an Irish Medical Missionary of Mary doctor, Sr Maura O'Donoghue, detailing the abuse and rape of nuns by priests and bishops in various African countries. The nuns who became pregnant were sent for abortions by their rapists, while those guilty of the abuse were portrayed as victims of 'seductive temptresses'. Sr O'Donoghue's report was given to the Vatican, and there, unsurprisingly, it rested. Such a mind-set, where women are treated as second-class citizens, is the very one that, in my opinion, resulted in the Eighth Amendment. Here was the same Church, in alliance in 1983 with conservative Catholic doctors and supine politicians in order to change our Constitution to restrict women's reproductive rights, while at the same time abusing vulnerable women and pushing those they had raped to have abortions. The hypocrisy was stunning.

With repeal of the Eighth in mind, in September 2014 I decided to stand for election to the position of chairman of the Institute of Obstetricians and Gynaecologists (IOG). The Institute is a constituent faculty of the Royal College of Physicians in Ireland and is responsible for training specialists in obstetrics/gynaecology and also has a role in lobbying to improve women's healthcare. Given the focus on maternity care and the Eighth Amendment, which was only likely to grow over the coming years, I believed the Institute should have a leading role in educating and advising the public and politicians about the issues involved. I could not be sure, but I calculated that there was a fair possibility that a referendum to change or repeal the Eighth Amendment might take place during the three-year term of the incoming chairman, therefore giving me a voice that I wouldn't have otherwise. No one else stood for election, so I duly became the chairman-elect. My term of office would commence the following September.*

Before the end of 2014 I was involved in one of the most distressing situations I have experienced in my entire medical career. In early December I took a call from a solicitor who wanted me to give an

---

*In fact I started in May 2015.

expert opinion on a case that she flagged as likely to be very controversial. *Here we go again*, I thought to myself, as she explained the background. A pregnant woman in her mid twenties, Miss P, the mother of two small children, aged four and six, had suffered catastrophic irreversible brain injury as a result of a cyst in her brain. She was on a ventilator and had been receiving maternal somatic support in a hospital outside Dublin (maternal somatic support refers to life support of a pregnant woman's body after brain death has been confirmed so the fetus can be delivered). She was fifteen weeks pregnant. Her father gave evidence at her inquest that the family were told on 29 November that 'the [fetal] heartbeat was still there and under the Constitution the medical staff had to put her on a life support machine.'

Miss P was transferred to Beaumont Hospital in Dublin in the early hours of Sunday, 30 November. The next day the medical team sought legal advice about what they should do next. The doctors were concerned that because of the Eighth Amendment, they could not stop somatic support and were obliged to try to keep the pregnancy going in order to vindicate the 'equal right to life' of the fetus. The multidisciplinary team met again on Tuesday, 2 December. A note in Miss P's hospital chart following the meeting captures the doctors' uncertainty. They were 'still waiting for legal issues with fetal rights, team will come back within 48 hours. They will bring it to the higher court.' On 3 December an angiogram was performed that showed no blood flow to the brain. Miss P's death was recorded at 5.20 p.m., and staff prepared to inform her family.

The consultant neurosurgeon, however, then told the family that because there was significant legal uncertainty, a meeting would now take place in the CEO's office with the legal team. In my evidence to the inquest I noted that the following day, 4 December, 'the family were spoken to at length about the interpretation of Irish constitutional law . . . there were difficulties from a legal point of view surrounding the Constitution.' The medical team made the decision to continue with somatic support and to transfer Miss P's body back to the original hospital as soon as a bed became available. This took place on Monday, 8 December.

She would have had to be kept on life support for several months in what would be pushing experimental medicine to the limits.

Although there are reports in the world literature of successful out-comes of pregnancy in such circumstances, there are none in pregnancies as early as Miss P's. The hospital notes record repeatedly that the family were distressed by what was happening. The only remedy for Miss P's father was to take a case against the HSE to see if life support could be discontinued in order to allow his daughter to complete her death with dignity.

Two days before Christmas the case went to the High Court, where all the pomp and legal muscle that such a setting implies were very much in evidence. There were eleven barristers in the court – three representing the family of Miss P, three more for the HSE, two for the deceased woman herself, two for the interests of the fetus, and one for the hospital. The case was heard before the president of the High Court, Mr Justice Nicholas Kearns, accompanied by Ms Justice Marie Baker and Ms Justice Caroline Costello.

The question before the court was whether it was 'practicable' to vindicate the right to life of the unborn as provided for in the Eighth Amendment by attaching the young woman's organs to machines in an experiment to see if her fetus could be delivered some weeks in the future. Her family pleaded for her to be let go with dignity.

The court heard very upsetting evidence about the condition of Miss P's body, in particular the fact that she was almost unrecogniz-able because of tissue swelling, and that there was fluid leaking from a scar in her skull where a drain had been placed in an attempt to reduce pressure on her brain. Particularly disturbing was the descrip-tion of her young children being brought to see their dead mother for the last time. The nurses had applied make-up to Miss P's eyes in an effort to hide what was happening, but her eyes were so swollen with gelatinous material oozing from them that they couldn't be closed. Her children were deeply distressed.

Medical witnesses, myself included, repeatedly described the treat-ment Miss P was receiving as experimental, given the specific circumstances of the case. Dr Peter McKenna, former master of the Rotunda Hospital, described continuation of her care as 'going from the extraordinary to the grotesque'. I agreed, 100 per cent.

I appeared as a witness for the family. I gave evidence that there was little prospect of the fetus reaching viability, and that I had found only three cases in world literature where maternal somatic support begun before eighteen weeks had had a successful outcome. There was also a risk of infection to the unborn. 'Just because something can be done in medicine, does not mean it should be,' I said. In my view, I told the court, the most ethical approach would be to adhere to the next-of-kin's wishes.

I told the court that 'we are unclear as to what we [doctors] can do in this country as a consequence of the Eighth Amendment. It puts us in a very difficult position and we are not legally qualified to make those decisions, so we are guided by the courts, which is why we are here.' Asked by Justice Kearns if medical or legal guidelines would be helpful, I replied that the removal of the Eighth would be even more helpful.

The hearing lasted all day on Tuesday, 23 December, and on the following day, Christmas Eve, legal submissions were made to the judges. Christmas Day was a sombre affair in our home that year as we thought of the agony of Miss P's family.

On Stephen's Day, the judges reached their decision: Miss P could be laid to rest by her family. This was not a case of abortion, they held, with the entire medical evidence showing that the 'prospects for a successful delivery of a live baby in this case are virtually non-existent'.

I found the judges' argument rather Jesuitical – if the case was not about abortion, then the Eighth Amendment was not relevant. Clearly it was the doctors' understanding of the Eighth Amendment that had caused them to fear that if they turned off Miss P's life support, they could be accused of performing an illegal termination of pregnancy. I was disappointed that the High Court had not engaged with the impact of the Eighth Amendment on medical practice.

As we entered 2015, increasing efforts were being made to get repeal of the Eighth on to the political agenda. I thought it interesting that in the middle of December Leo Varadkar, Minister for Health since July, had made a significant speech in the Dáil, identifying the existing abortion laws as 'too restrictive' and having a 'chilling effect' on doctors. However, Enda Kenny ruled out a referendum in the lifetime of his government.

In January 2015 I worked with Amnesty International on its report *She is Not a Criminal: The Impact of Ireland's Abortion Law*, which was published later that year, and in October, along with three other doctors from countries with restrictive abortion laws, I spoke on an Amnesty-convened panel at an International Federation of Obstetrics and Gynaecology conference in Vancouver.

Professor Chafik Chraïbi spoke about the situation in Morocco, where, after a thirty-year career, he had been sacked from his position at the Maternité des Orangers hospital in Rabat earlier in the year. With around 4,500 deaths annually due to unsafe abortion, he had invited in a film crew for a television documentary on Morocco's restrictive abortion laws, which only allowed termination in the case of a threat to the woman's life or health. His sacking caused a public furore, and King Mohammed VI ordered the government to review abortion law.*

Dr Guillermo Ortiz Avendaño, from the Woman's National Hospital in El Salvador, addressed the lethal impact of the total ban on abortion in his country, where criminal prosecutions of women and doctors are common. Reports from El Salvador make it clear that, as well as dying from clandestine abortion, women also die after being refused medical treatment. Some doctors, for example, will not give chemotherapy to a pregnant woman with cancer for fear of harming the fetus. Others allow ectopic pregnancies to continue until the woman's fallopian tube ruptures, because they fear that even these embryos growing outside the womb will be considered living beings under the strict law. Nearly 40 per cent of maternal deaths in El Salvador are of teenage girls who kill themselves because they are distraught over their pregnancies. The laws are so strict that well over a hundred women who have had miscarriages have been reported to police as having had abortions, charged with homicide and sent to prison.

Meanwhile, Dr Aníbal Faúndes, emeritus professor of obstetrics at the State University of Campinas in Brazil, spoke about the estimated 250,000 women who are hospitalized from complications from abortions annually, and the 200 women or more who die. If women are hospitalized, they can be reported to the police by their doctors. Several hundred criminal cases are registered against women in Brazil each year.

* In June 2016 Morocco would amend its law to provide for legal abortion, beyond risk to health and life, in cases of rape or incest and fetal abnormalities.

When it came to my turn, I spoke about the historical background of the near-total ban on abortion in Ireland, observing that Ireland had been a *de facto* theocracy after independence in 1922, when the new state ceded control of education and health to the Catholic Church. I talked about the Eighth Amendment and the subsequent amendments that enshrined hypocrisy in the Constitution. I went through Savita's case and the Irish alphabet of tragic cases that define the impact of the Eighth. Luckily, I told them, women in Ireland had the escape valve of the UK and generally most women had the means to travel. However, as with Morocco, El Salvador and Brazil, poor and marginalized women suffered most.

As part of the 2015 campaign, Amnesty International published a letter by 838 doctors in forty-four countries calling for the decriminalization of abortion. Alongside doctors from Africa, Asia and South America, several Irish GPs and consultants, including myself, put our names to the letter. Criminalization 'prevents healthcare providers from delivering timely, medically indicated care in accordance with their patients' wishes', the letter said. 'It impedes and disregards sound medical judgement and can undermine the professional duty of care and confidentiality that doctors bear towards their patients.'

As Institute chairperson, I was asked for a comment on publication of the Amnesty letter. I said that Irish medical staff faced a 'legal and ethical tightrope' and repeated that under the current law 'we must wait until women become sick enough before we can intervene. How close to death do you have to be? There is no answer to that.'

On 3 October 2015 *Irish Times* journalist Kitty Holland published a report on the growing number of women in Ireland who were importing 'abortion pills' from outside the state. She took the case study of 'Emily', who had imported mifepristone and misoprostol from a Netherlands-based NGO that posts pills to women all over the world. She paid €90 for the pills, which arrived within two weeks. Emily experienced severe pain and vomiting and continued to bleed for two weeks after the termination.

The story brought vividly into the public domain an issue that was of increasing concern: the illegal importation of abortion pills in Ireland and the serious medical consequences that could arise. As chair of the IOG, I warned about the dangers of taking medication without proper medical consultation.

Three weeks later, in a move that echoed the Irish Women's Liberation Movement's famous contraceptive train of 1971,* an 'abortion pill bus', organized by the campaign group Reproductive Rights against Oppression, Sexism and Austerity (ROSA), set off from Dublin on a two-day tour across Ireland, carrying abortion pills and information on how Irish women could access abortions. Again, having a voice because of my role as chair of the Institute, I commented that if any woman had problems after taking such tablets, she would be well looked after if she went to one of our hospitals. I wanted to signal to women that they could seek medical help if problems arose. While I could reassure women about the care they would receive in our hospitals, I could not guarantee that they would not be in legal trouble, given that in Northern Ireland the previous year a nineteen-year-old woman bought abortion pills online, took them and then miscarried. Eight days later her housemates reported her to the police and she was arrested.†

At the end of 2015 Taoiseach Enda Kenny announced that if Fine Gael was returned to government following the imminent general election, the question of the Eighth Amendment would be the first issue considered by the planned Citizens' Assembly, a body comprising ninety-nine representative citizens, chosen at random, with a chair, and an advisory group to provide impartial advice. The Citizens' Assembly was planned as an exercise in 'deliberative democracy',

---

*Contraception was still illegal in Ireland in the early seventies. In May 1971 forty-seven members of the IWLM took the train to Belfast with the intention of buying contraceptives, bringing them back to Dublin and putting the Irish authorities on the spot. However, until they reached the pharmacy in Belfast they did not realize that women required a prescription for many forms of contraception, including the pill. Not wanting to return to Dublin waving fistfuls of condoms (thereby focusing minds on male genitalia), one of their number, journalist Nell McCafferty, had the inspired idea of buying hundreds of packets of aspirin and simply pretending they were contraceptive pills. The women's return to Connolly, brandishing 'the pill', as well as condoms and spermicidal jelly, was a media sensation. Asked by customs officers if they had anything to declare, they made it clear that they had all manner of forbidden contraceptives. The customs men were befuddled, took no action and the women left the station in triumph, having made their point that the law was ridiculous.

† In April 2016 Belfast Crown Court sentenced her to three months in prison, suspended for two years, under the 1861 Offences Against the Person Act.

a process in which the public deliberation of representative citizens can assist legislators on difficult political and social issues by distilling authentic public opinion, independent of political bias. The Assembly would hear presentations from experts and interested parties on five key policy issues facing Ireland, the Eighth Amendment being the first of these, discuss and consider what they heard, and then come up with recommendations to the Oireachtas.

After so many years of inaction on the Eighth, many suspected this was a classic politician's ploy to kick the can further down the road (perhaps so far down the road that it would be a problem for a subsequent administration). But whatever the government and activists anticipated or feared, everyone was in for quite a surprise.

Retired Supreme Court judge Mary Laffoy was appointed chairperson of the Citizens' Assembly in July 2016, and its first working meeting was held in late November. On the Assembly's advisory group to provide impartial advice on medical, legal and ethical issues regarding the Eighth Amendment were two obstetricians, Elizabeth Dunn, a consultant at Wexford Hospital, and Declan Keane, a consultant and former master at the NMH; two constitutional lawyers, Rachel Walsh and Oran Doyle, and Deirdre Madden, an expert in medical law and ethics.

Over four weekends the Assembly heard from a wide variety of medical, legal and policy experts. All along the Assembly had been receiving submissions from individuals and advocacy groups, and, based on feedback from members, the chairperson selected seventeen organizations to make presentations: Amnesty International Ireland, Atheist Ireland, Coalition to Repeal the Eighth Amendment, Doctors for Choice, Doctors for Life Ireland, Every Life Counts, Family and Life, the Irish Catholic Bishops' Conference, the Irish Family Planning Association, Parents for Choice, the Pro Life Campaign, the General Synod of the Church of Ireland, the Iona Institute, the National Women's Council of Ireland, the Union of Students in Ireland, Women Hurt and Youth Defence. These presentations were the final contributions the participants heard prior to assembling for a fifth weekend to decide on their recommendations to the Oireachtas.

Though the Pro Life Campaign attempted to undermine the Assembly from the outset, dubbing it a 'pretend process with a prearranged outcome' and vowing to 'challenge this sham process every step of the way', no one could reasonably accuse the Assembly of not inviting and listening to the full spectrum of opinion.★

The proceedings were live-streamed and I watched them closely. I had no contact or involvement with the Citizens' Assembly itself, but I was hopeful that the Assembly would conclude, based on all the evidence being presented, that the Eighth Amendment was indeed harmful and needed to be removed from the Constitution.

On Saturday, 22 April 2017, the Citizens' Assembly held three votes on Article 40.3.3 of the Constitution, the Eighth Amendment. The first held that it should not be retained in full (79 votes to 12). The second recommended that it should be replaced or amended (50 votes) rather than deleted and not replaced (39 votes). And the final vote on Saturday was a majority (51 votes) for the Oireachtas legislating regarding 'termination of pregnancy, any rights of the unborn, and any rights of the pregnant woman' rather than making direct provisions within the Constitution itself (38 votes).

On the Sunday, the Assembly voted on a range of thirteen potential circumstances in which abortion might be permitted, ranging from 'Real and substantial physical risk to the life of the woman' to 'No restriction as to reasons'. For each one of these thirteen scenarios the Assembly voted by a majority that abortion should be permitted. That they were in favour of permitting abortion when there was a real and substantial risk to a woman's life (99 per cent) was perhaps not so surprising. But that they voted so strongly (64 per cent) in favour of permitting abortion without restriction as to reasons was startling. The conclusions of the Citizens' Assembly transformed the debate on abortion in Ireland – the Eighth Amendment was now a live political issue.

★ All of the Citizens' Assembly's work on the Eighth Amendment and the other topics it considered can be viewed on the website www.citizensassembly.ie and presentations and proceedings are available on its YouTube channel.

11.   Falling down a rabbit hole

Another live political issue at this time – one that had just as profound implications for women's health as the Eighth Amendment – had flared up unexpectedly in the period before and after my retirement in December 2016. For me, the issue was not just a matter of public policy, but concerned an institution I love, the National Maternity Hospital. After a career of more than three decades at Holles Street, I found myself at the heart of the very public controversy over the plan to relocate the hospital to the campus of St Vincent's Hospital. The series of events that unfolded made me wonder if, like Alice in Wonderland, I had fallen through a rabbit hole into a place where logic was turned on its head. The episode had many tortuous twists and turns, and is not yet resolved.

When it comes to the medical care of women, I believe in two fundamental principles. First, that maternity hospitals need their own governance and budgetary independence, and, second, that religious teaching or belief should have no role in determining the care given to women. It is my belief in these two principles that brought me into direct conflict over the relocation plan.

It was not relocation itself that gave me any difficulty. Plans had been drawn up for a superb new hospital that would offer state-of-the-art facilities for mothers and infants, in contrast to the cramped 1930s buildings on Holles Street in the centre of Dublin. However, over the course of 2015 and 2016, it became obvious that both principles – independence and freedom from a religious ethos – were in severe jeopardy.

In my decades of clinical experience I have seen at first hand the pitfalls and dangers of integrating maternity units into general hospitals. In the past few years alone I have chaired and contributed to review teams, and written expert reports, following adverse incidents that have tragically included maternal and infant deaths in Galway, Portiuncula, Sligo, Cavan, Drogheda and Portlaoise. In all of these cases, the governance of maternity services came under that of the general hospital.

The 2016 National Maternity Strategy was developed to 'provide the framework for a new and better maternity service' in response to these incidents, with particular emphasis given to the report into the death of Savita Halappanavar in Galway in 2012. Among the key recommendations are that all stand-alone maternity hospitals be co-located with an adult acute hospital, and that the mastership model of management be continued, since it provides a sound governance model. Under this model day-to-day operational control of the hospital rests with a master, an obstetrician and gynaecologist elected by the hospital's governors – so that effectively the hospital's CEO is also a working doctor. This approach combines responsibility with accountability, and a unique clinical knowledge of the business of childbirth. When maternity services are just another part of a general hospital, they lose out on having that specialized knowledge.

I have worked in Dublin, London and Houston, and have spoken at and attended conferences around the world, meeting and talking with international colleagues. It could not be clearer to me that hospitals operated under a religious ethos restrict women's reproductive healthcare. Catholic ethos is the issue in Ireland, and in all Catholic hospitals around the world the provision of healthcare is subject to 'Ethical and Research Directives' issued by the local national bishops' conferences or councils, but founded on the universal underlying principles of Catholic teaching and canon law. There is thus a prohibition on contraception or sterilization for the purposes of preventing pregnancy, abortion (including the early delivery of non-viable pregnancies), assisted fertility treatments such as IVF, some genetic testing and gender-reassignment surgery. Failure to comply with the directives is a violation of canon law.

Furthermore, any land owned by a religious order is 'ecclesiastical land', and any hospital or healthcare facility built on that land must adhere to canon law. The property and land owned by Catholic organizations is subject to 'Vatican Guidelines for the Administration of Assets in Institutes of Consecrated Life and Society's Apostolic Life', the most recent version of which was published in 2014. This point about land is critical: Catholic ethos must apply to any healthcare facility built on Catholic land, *irrespective of the ownership of any individual buildings.*

If we look around the world, there are multiple examples of the impact of Catholic Church involvement in maternity and gynae-cology services.

In the US Catholic hospitals must comply with 'The Ethical and Religious Directives for Catholic Healthcare Services' issued by America's Conference of Catholic Bishops. These prohibit a range of reproductive healthcare services, even when a woman's life or health is in danger (a similar directive is issued by Irish bishops). In 2009 Sr Margaret McBride, an administrator at St Joseph's Hospital and Medical Center in Phoenix, Arizona, was excommunicated by the bishop of Phoenix because she had agreed to an abortion for a 27-year-old woman who was eleven weeks pregnant with her fifth child. The woman's hospital chart noted 'right heart failure', and her doctors told her that if she continued with the pregnancy, her risk of mortality was 'close to 100 per cent'.

Professor Lisa Sowle Cahill, a theologian and ethicist at Boston College, described the dilemma later: 'There was no good way out of it. The official Church position would mandate that the correct solution would be to let both the mother and the child die.'

In 2016 the American Civil Liberties Union (ACLU) published the report *Health Care Denied*, which included numerous first-hand accounts of women who did not receive appropriate medical care in faith-based hospitals in the US. The report found one in six hospital beds in the US is in a facility that complies with the Catholic bishops' directives, and that in some states more than 40 per cent of all hospital beds are in a Catholic-run facility, leaving entire regions without any option for certain reproductive healthcare services, despite being funded each year by billions of taxpayers' dollars.

In 2008 the archbishop of Westminster, Cardinal Cormac Murphy-O'Connor, sacked the entire board of the private Catholic St John and St Elizabeth Hospital in London following disputes over staff support for contraception, abortion and gender-reassignment surgery. The cardinal had appointed an auxiliary bishop of Westminster to the hospital's ethics committee to ensure its adherence to Catholic teaching the previous year, and in December 2007 two of the hospital's directors resigned in protest, saying the cardinal 'placed Catholic values above patient care'.

In a 2012 radio interview, Dr Bernadette White, clinical director of the Mercy Maternity Hospital in Melbourne, addressed the clinical situation that resulted in the death of Savita Halappanavar in Ireland. She said that in a similar clinical scenario in her hospital, 5 per cent of women were prepared to accept the associated risks, while the remaining 95 per cent who requested a termination were transferred out to a non-Catholic hospital.

A woman developing sepsis requires immediate treatment, and it is poor clinical practice for physicians to delay treatment while they phone around the city or state in search of a hospital that will accept her. That is the reality, however, of what happens in Australia's Catholic hospitals, even though termination of pregnancy is legal in Australia.

Like many twentieth-century hospitals, as birth numbers increased, the NMH outgrew its Holles Street premises. When the current building opened in 1938, a little over 2,000 women gave birth in the hospital. Sixty years later, in the last year of my mastership, 7,682 babies were born in Holles Street, and population trends in Dublin were such that the number would continue to increase. In my final clinical report I said there was 'urgent need for significant capital investment in the infrastructure of the hospital'.

I recall chatting with future Taoiseach Enda Kenny in the hospital after the birth of one of his children. At the time he was a TD, and I jokingly said to him that when he became Minister for Health he was to make sure we got a new hospital.

From the early 2000s there was a clear understanding among successive masters not only that there was an urgent need for a new hospital, but that it should be co-located with a general hospital. By the end of 2000 my successor, Declan Keane, reported that '[T]he long-term infrastructural needs of the hospital will now probably be best served by moving to an alternative site, which will most likely be St Vincent's Hospital.' In his final report, for 2004, Dr Keane recorded that in his seven years in the job, the NMH had been met by 'masterly inactivity and profound procrastination' when it came to planning for a new hospital.

In his first annual report the following year the new master, Michael Robson, described the infrastructure of the hospital as 'totally inadequate' and expressed the hope that the forthcoming review of maternity services in the Greater Dublin Area would confirm the suitability of the St Vincent's campus for a new NMH.

In May 2007 the Department of Health and HSE commissioned KPMG to conduct a 'Review of Maternity and Gynaecology Services in the Greater Dublin Area'. It was completed in August 2008. A key observation of the report noted that it was 'well recognised that for optimal clinical outcome, maternity services should be co-located with acute adult services, or in the case of neonatology and fetal medicine be tri-located with adult and paediatric services'.

Co-location has a specific meaning in a healthcare context: it is where separate hospitals co-exist on the same footprint under separate governance arrangements, but sharing support services. This is particularly desirable when hospitals providing specialist services are located alongside general hospitals. St James's Hospital, for instance, hosts St Luke's and the Jonathan Swift Clinic on its campus and will host the new National Paediatric Hospital. When it comes to maternity care, co-location is vital. Many of the problems that have arisen in our maternity services have been in units that are integrated into, rather than co-located with, general hospitals. In such set-ups maternity care comes down the list of priorities. Midwives get reassigned to surgical or medical wards, operating theatres are used for non-obstetrical or gynaecological procedures, and operating lists are disproportionately cancelled.

The KPMG report recommended that two of the three maternity hospitals in Dublin should be co-located with an adult hospital, and one should be tri-located with the planned National Paediatric Hospital. St Vincent's Hospital had 'demonstrated willingness to accommodate a maternity hospital on site', and the recommendation, therefore, was that the Coombe Hospital should move to Tallaght, the NMH should move to St Vincent's, and the Rotunda should move to the Mater Hospital, since that was the chosen location, at that time, for the new National Paediatric Hospital.

The worldwide financial crisis that followed the collapse of Lehman Brothers in September 2008 changed everything. The Irish economy went into freefall. By the time the government made a formal request for financial support from the European Union Financial Stability Fund and the International Monetary Fund (IMF) in November 2010 – the Troika bailout – it was clear that in the short term there were no funds available for large capital projects.

★

Rhona Mahony began her term as master on 1 January 2012. In her first clinical report she recorded that over 9,100 babies had been born in her first year, with an average of 25 per day, but on three days in the year more than 40 babies had been delivered. She noted that she had been 'frequently quoted in my belief that NMH needs to be housed in a modern fit for purpose facility co-located with a general hospital', although no specific reference was made to St Vincent's. In the background there had been real hope during the year for a new hospital sooner rather than later.

Perhaps ironically, the activity of the National Asset Management Agency (NAMA) – a body set up in the wake of the banking crisis – seemed to offer an opportunity for progress at last. In 2012 the Department of Health, the HSE and the NMH had agreed the new maternity hospital would occupy the two front blocks of a new building on the Elm Park business campus on Merrion Road. It was close to St Vincent's in a building already constructed, part of a development formerly owned by the developers Bernard McNamara and Jerry O'Reilly, but then in receivership and controlled by NAMA.

A portion of this had been earmarked in its planning permission for a private day care hospital that hadn't gone ahead. The new plan for the NMH, however, was abandoned the day before an agreement was to be signed, because the Irish Development Agency (IDA) wanted the building for Novartis, a Swiss pharmaceutical multinational, and one of its foreign direct investment clients. Labour Party Senator Kevin Humphries, a board member of the NMH at the time, said in 2017 that '[I]t seemed to be all go', to the extent that planning permission was supposed to be lodged. The then Minister for Health, James Reilly, later confirmed that '[W]e [the Department of Health] certainly had an interest in it and thought "That's great, it's so near to St Vincent's Hospital." But then the IDA stepped in and they wanted it. They had a client that was going to bring 1,000 jobs. The decision was made by NAMA ultimately.'

I have been told by people involved that the Department of Health had been prepared to offer €50 million for the site, but the IDA offered €100 million, and that Michael Noonan, Minister for Finance, had the final say.

It was not, therefore, until 27 May 2013 that James Reilly could announce the government's intention to relocate the National Maternity Hospital to St Vincent's Elm Park campus. An indicative sum of €150 million was approved in the HSE's Capital Plan for the project.

It could not have been clearer that the ambition of both hospitals was co-location. Welcoming the announcement, the CEO of St Vincent's Healthcare Group (SVHG), Nicky Jermyn, observed that the SVHG and the NMH 'currently enjoy a very close working relationship'. He added that '[O]ver the years many clinical synergies have been created in anticipation of co-location. We look forward to closer physical proximity and enhanced collaboration in the best interest of patients.' Meanwhile, Professor Noel Whelan, chairman of St Vincent's, and a board member for some twenty-six years, was a major supporter of co-location.

Negotiations and planning with St Vincent's proceeded amicably for a year. An outline feasibility study for the co-location was carried out by Scott Tallon Walker Architects in 2013, and a project board was established in July of that year to oversee the development. It included representatives from the NMH, SVHG, the Department of Health, HSE, the National Clinical Programme in Obstetrics and Gynaecology, and the National Clinical Programme in Paediatrics and Neonatology.

On 13 May 2014 Minister Reilly announced that contracts had been signed with a team of architects, surveyors and engineers. The final design of the building was by O'Connell Mahon Architects, and the principal linkage with the SVHG hospital was by way of a corridor connecting the operating theatres of St Vincent's public hospital with the new NMH. Construction would commence in 2016, with an expected completion date in 2019. It appeared, finally, to be all systems go.

Even before the Minister's optimistic announcement in May 2014, problems with the co-location project had already emerged. And these would deepen as the year went on.

On Thursday, 16 January 2014, there had been a stormy meeting between senior figures at SVHG and the Oireachtas Public Accounts Committee (PAC), an encounter that would play out with consequences for the NMH move. The issue of salary 'top-ups' paid to senior administrators from some thirty-four 'Section 38' organizations,* including hospitals, had been a major and controversial national issue towards the end of 2013. St Vincent's had attracted sharp political criticism for refusing initially to release information to the PAC in December, by which time all other hospitals had made disclosures. It finally changed course, and late on 23 December it disclosed that Nicky Jermyn, CEO of the public hospital since April 1994 and CEO of SVHG from its establishment in January 2003, was receiving €136,591 in addition to his HSE-funded salary of €136,282, plus a car allowance of around €20,000. At the January PAC meeting members accused St Vincent's of being non-compliant with public sector pay policy, in particular with regard to Jermyn's remuneration.

Jermyn and Noel Whelan were joined at the PAC meeting by James Menton (a former senior partner of KPMG), the chair of SVHG's finance committee, Stewart Harrington, its deputy chairman, and Thomas Lynch, a non-executive director and chair of both the Ireland East Hospital Group† and the Mater Hospital. In their submission to the PAC, St Vincent's recorded that SVHG Ltd was a private company guaranteed by shares whose sole shareholders were the Religious Sisters of Charity. The two hospitals – private and public – at Elm Park 'are on private land owned by the [Sisters of Charity]'.

Deputy Simon Harris, a Fine Gael member of the PAC, acknowledged the 'excellent service' SVHG provided to patients, and said he was very happy to put it on the record that he believed that no charitable funds had been used for pay or pensions. However, Harris said that he was concerned that '[T]he conclusion of the report from the Comptroller and Auditor General is that St Vincent's pledged publicly funded assets in return for bank finance for the development of its private hospital', opened in November 2010.

What Simon Harris was referring to was that SVHG had entered into several mortgage arrangements with Bank of Ireland in 2009 and 2010. Of particular note was the arrangement undertaken in October 2010 that gave Bank of Ireland 'a fixed charge over the entire

---

* Section 38 organizations provide health or personal social services on behalf of the HSE.

† One of the seven groupings under which the HSE administers hospitals.

St Vincent's Hospital site' and 'a floating charge over all the under-taking, property and assets of SVHG both present and future'. This was a sore point with the HSE.

In 2004 the old Eastern Regional Health Authority had made a €200 million grant for a clinic and science building to St Vincent's, but in an oversight had omitted to secure the funded assets in favour of the state through a legal security agreement, although this was later rectified. Asked by Harris if 'the hospital board [had] any duty or responsibility in terms of taxpayers' assets', Stewart Harrington replied, 'I do not believe so.' The HSE and the Department of Health thought otherwise, given the level of funding each year to St Vincent's, including capital expenditure.

As the hearing continued, it became clear that St Vincent's, which had received about €220 million of funding from the HSE in 2012 to provide services in its public hospitals (St Vincent's and St Michael's in Dun Laoghaire), had been of the view, based on legal advice, that they were fully compliant with public sector pay policy. Professor Whelan acknowledged that, while '[t]echnically we were compliant, in the public interest we would say we wish to go into compliance now'.

The issue for the PAC was Nicky Jermyn's dual role in both the private and public hospitals, with a total remuneration twice his public sector salary. They wanted to know, as Chairman John McGuinness expressed it, 'how Mr Jermyn's private work and public work are costed and if both are kept separate. Is there confusion in the handling of patients between the public and private hospitals? Are patients referred to the private hospital for income?'

James Menton then confirmed to the PAC what was widespread knowledge in medical circles: that the private hospital was losing money, having made a loss of €10.86 million in 2012, a 20 per cent increase on the previous year's loss.

As a consequence of the PAC hearing, Jermyn stepped down from his dual role, and Professor Michael Keane, a practising clinician, was appointed CEO of the public hospital.

With his decades of service to the state, Noel Whelan understood and accepted the point at which state funding and voluntary hospitals intersect. As it would turn out, not all his board colleagues agreed with him, and his removal from the SVHG board was swift and brutal. In September 2014 he was called to a special meeting at

St Vincent's, where he was informed that his resignation was immediately required. He was being replaced by James Menton. This was a return to the board for Menton, who had previously stood down in disagreement with the board's acceptance that the state had an oversight role in the compliance of SVHG, given its level of state funding. As Whelan departed, the two Sisters of Charity on the board wept.

Whelan's removal was part of a wholesale restructuring of the St Vincent's board in 2014. In total six members retired or resigned by the end of the year. As well as Professor Whelan, Stewart Harrington and Dr Michael Somers, former head of the National Treasury Management Agency, also departed. The appointment of six new directors was announced on 9 January 2015.

During the final months of 2014 St Vincent's position in respect of the new NMH underwent a complete turnaround, and the question of clinical and corporate governance now became a sticking point in negotiations.

St Vincent's said that Holles Street could locate the new maternity hospital on its grounds only if the NMH became a branch of its healthcare group, under SVHG corporate and clinical control, with a single governance system for the entire campus, i.e., the complete integration of the NMH into SVHG, effectively making it the maternity wing of the general hospital.

A project timeline that was circulated to NMH doctors in 2016 records how Holles Street viewed matters in 2014. The entry for November 2014 reads: 'Dramatic change in composition of SVHG Board and new Chairman. The rules of engagement change and SVHG impose a series of new requirements for this project to proceed. These requirements include the dissolution of the NMH.'

The NMH had been taken completely by surprise, as journalist Dearbhail McDonald reported in the *Sunday Independent* in 2016, 'as it had always intended to transfer to St Vincent's as a stand-alone entity with responsibility for its clinical and commercial outcomes. "There was never any discussion of a complete take-over until then," said one person familiar with the negotiations. "Had there been, it would have been a red line from the very start." '

Of course it would. The NMH had a long tradition of self-governance, based on the mastership model, and the Catholic ethos of St Vincent's meant that co-location was the only way to maintain independence of medical practice.

Nonetheless, in January 2015, negotiations continued, albeit without a meeting of minds. In March a joint project board and project team meeting was held, during which the design team made a presentation 'to address stated concerns by SVHG in relation to clinical linkages and technical design planning issues'.

Speaking to the Dáil's PAC that April, Tony O'Brien, HSE's director general, characterized the St Vincent's private hospital's relationship to the public hospital as one of 'parasitic dependence'. He expressed concern that the private hospital was being run off the back of the public one, and indicated that the HSE might have to consider the issue of special administration for St Vincent's if the hospital was not forthcoming on the issue of consultants admitting patients to the private hospital without, in the HSE's view, the contractual rights to do so.

O'Brien had concerns about overall governance issues and noted that Noel Whelan, who had given the undertaking to become compliant with public sector pay policy, had made some important progress 'before his removal from office by the group's shareholders'. He said the HSE was coming close to the stage where it could not accept the situation any more in relation to corporate governance at SVHG.

His comments to the PAC caused fury at St Vincent's. Later that day the CEO, Professor Keane, wrote to senior officials in the HSE, stating that, because of O'Brien's remarks, St Vincent's would not be able to attend an imminent project board meeting, or any other meetings regarding the relocation of the NMH, until further notice. It would be another three months before St Vincent's re-engaged with the project.

In December the project board confirmed that it was satisfied that the design was ready for submission to An Bord Pleanála but said that 'on the foot of outstanding governance issues' SVHG was declining to issue the required letter of consent so that the application could be submitted.

St Vincent's were holding firm in their demands for complete control of the NMH, and their refusal to issue the letter now stalled the project once more. Even the direct intervention of Leo Varadkar, the then Minister for Health, failed to break the deadlock.

Minister Varadkar was fully in favour of co-location, and unhappy with St Vincent's position, so much so that he had made a surprise appearance at a meeting between the two hospitals towards the end of 2015, to tell the St Vincent's team that his department wanted co-location rather than integration, as proposed by St Vincent's. He was met with a complete refusal to shift position.

I was astounded when I heard about St Vincent's response to Minister Varadkar. NMH representatives described its attitude as contemptuous, even aggressive, and certainly disrespectful. I have had many robust exchanges with successive ministers, but they were always conducted with respect for the person and the office, and with the understanding that the Minister controls state funding. Yet here was St Vincent's, under intense pressure from the Minister, his department and the HSE, strangely impervious to the normal give and take of such a negotiation process.

In January 2016, and with my support, Rhona Mahony embarked on a new approach to persuade the Department of Health, the HSE and the public of the merits of Holles Street's position. In her 2015 annual report, delivered in late January, she argued that 'it is vital that tertiary maternity and neonatal services and expertise are not subjugated to adult services which have different and competing requirements.'

In early February I chaired a workshop in Trinity College's Long Room Hub, organized by the School of English and Department of History, entitled 'Medicine, Health and Welfare'. The workshop was part of Trinity's ongoing 'Institutions and Ireland' series. A group of scholars looked at a number of historically difficult matters such as maternal and infant mortality, Magdalene Laundries, infanticide, the history of concealed pregnancy, and the practice of burying still-born babies or those born out of wedlock in *cillíní*.* It was a timely reminder of the troubled history of Irish maternity services.

Dr Mahony gave the keynote speech, 'Birth of a Nation, 1916–2016', in which she criticized the 'profound influence' of the historic relationship between the Catholic Church and the state on female sexuality and reproductive health in Ireland in the first 100 years of the new state.

---

* Unconsecrated burial grounds.

Her remarks dovetailed with my own thinking. To my immense frustration, although I had been clinical director at the NMH from 2009 to 2014, I was not invited to join the ongoing negotiations with St Vincent's. From my perspective it seemed clear that the NMH team was on the back foot and needed to get a grip on what St Vincent's was trying to achieve if it was to more successfully fight our corner. Early in 2016 I had started to analyse the situation in greater depth.

What really puzzled me was why, or how, St Vincent's had remained so obdurate in the face of direct pressure from Minister Leo Varadkar, especially given the extent of their state funding.

Three issues seemed to me to be significant.

First, it was well known that the private hospital was loss-making. It had built too few theatres for its needs in the expectation that the public theatres could be used. Capacity in the public hospital made this impossible, so the private hospital was not viable. I knew that, since the NMH project had been mooted, many St Vincent's consultants were unhappy. They wanted the space earmarked for the NMH for building new theatres for their use. An obvious question arose: did the St Vincent's board want complete ownership of the NMH to solve their theatre capacity issue?

Second, it seemed obvious, too, given the financial woes of the private hospital and the outstanding loans with Bank of Ireland, that placing a new National Maternity Hospital with a probable value in excess of at least €150 million on its campus, and fully owned by SVHG, would undoubtedly strengthen the group's balance sheet and make future discussions with the banks a lot easier.

Increasingly, however, to the forefront of my mind came a third issue. Given that St Vincent's was a Catholic hospital and prohibited such procedures as vasectomy and tubal ligation, why would they even *want* to own a maternity hospital, especially now that the Protection of Life During Pregnancy Act permitted abortion in some cases, and the Eighth Amendment was firmly on the political agenda?

The NMH had developed a successful multidisciplinary reproductive medicine service in conjunction with the Merrion Fertility Clinic, and was currently the only teaching hospital in the country to have an assisted reproductive treatment service, another practice that was forbidden by Catholic teaching. Contraception, of course, was routinely prescribed, and abortion was provided in defined circumstances. So — again — *why did St Vincent's want to own a maternity hospital?*

Suddenly it occurred to me that I was perhaps looking at this conundrum the wrong way around. *What if St Vincent's wanted to control the NMH in order to have a fully Catholic maternity hospital in Ireland?* What if this was a deliberate move, in anticipation of the repeal of the Eighth Amendment, to establish in Ireland the kind of Catholic maternity hospital that operates in other countries?

I had no doubt that the Vatican was keeping a close eye on liberal developments in Ireland. The landmark passing of the referendum on same sex marriage in 2015 had provoked dismay and deep disquiet in Rome and in Irish Catholic circles. Abortion was clearly the next issue on the agenda. I had stood for election to the chair of the Institute of Obstetricians and Gynaecologists for the three-year term 2015 to 2018 precisely because I calculated that it was possible that a referendum might take place during my tenure, and I would therefore have a platform to argue in favour of repealing the Eighth Amendment.

Ireland, along with tiny Malta, was the only country in Europe that prohibited abortion in all cases, unless a woman's life was in danger. For conservative Catholics, retaining the Eighth Amendment in the Irish Constitution would be a last stand for the Church in Europe. And Ireland would be the field on which this major battle would be fought.

Adding to my concerns were developments in other Catholic-run hospitals, including the Mater in Dublin and in Cork. The Sisters of Mercy at the Mater had established a small committee, chaired by a senior member of the board, to put in train the transfer of their land to the Vatican. The sisters were elderly and their numbers were dwindling, and so a succession plan for the management of their assets was needed. That transfer into some kind of Vatican-controlled vehicle was now imminent and would effectively result in the land of the Sisters of Mercy being put outside the reach of the state 'in perpetuity'.

In March 2016 the paperwork was with Diarmuid Martin, the Catholic archbishop of Dublin. He had not signed it off, however, according to a member of the board of the Mater, who told me at the time that Martin 'sees the political implications' of such a move.

However, the bishop of Cork and Ross, John Buckley, had already signed off on the paperwork for the Sisters of Mercy in Cork to complete the transfer of ownership of their land. It seemed likely that the Sisters of Charity had begun to examine a similar transfer and did not want to encumber the land at Elm Park, as it would complicate or even prohibit any transaction. The NMH would be right in the middle of the campus.

In this respect I was mindful that St Vincent's is directly across the Merrion Road from the church of Our Lady Queen of Peace, which in 2008 transferred from the Archdiocese of Dublin to the Opus Dei Prelature. Opus Dei is a Catholic organization whose members are largely lay Catholics who put particular emphasis on serving God in their professional or working life. Secrecy is a major feature, and recruits are enjoined never to reveal their membership, adhering to Article 189 of the unpublished constitution: 'In order to achieve its aim more easily the Institute as such must live in concealment.'

Membership of Opus Dei in Ireland is not disclosed, but in 2011 its spokesman estimated it at around 700, including fifteen priests. Around 70 per cent of members are termed 'supernumeraries'. These are, typically, married men and women, and, although in theory they can come from any social group, in practice they are almost always senior figures in the professions, business and industry, such as lawyers, doctors, architects, engineers, bankers, accountants and company directors. Opus Dei members follow what is known as the 'Plan of Life', a daily regimen of prayer, meditation, an act of penance or mortification, and religious ceremonies. One key maxim is No. 627: 'Remain silent and you will never regret it, speak and you often will.' (Clearly not a maxim for life with which I agree.)

As I reflected on it, it was not inconceivable that Opus Dei might be taking an interest in the battle under way in the hospital just across the road from its Irish church. I had no way of knowing if any members of the board of St Vincent's were in Opus Dei, but there were many protagonists across a number of institutions and organizations who had an involvement with the NMH relocation project, and the ongoing impasse made sense if considered in the context of a conservative Catholic agenda. For me, the matter came into sharp focus and was straightforward. Based on all available evidence, with knowledge of the policy and practice at every Catholic hospital in the world without exception, it was clear that integration, rather than co-location, meant that the future NMH would not be able to operate as it did currently, and it would effectively become the maternity wing of St Vincent's, a Catholic hospital. It would no longer be able to function as a tertiary referral centre.

My experience with Savita had ensured that I never again wanted to hear the word 'Catholic' associated with anything to do with women's reproductive healthcare. Nor did I want to witness at least €150 million of taxpayers' money being effectively gifted to a private religious congregation. I simply could not accept this for the women of Ireland, or for the institution to which I had devoted most of my working life. It was time for a fresh offensive.

12.   A 'power grab' by St Vincent's

In March 2016, as St Vincent's still refused to re-engage with the NMH relocation project, Rhona Mahony asked if I would write to the key parties – the Minister for Health, the HSE, the boards of the NMH and SVHG – on behalf of the Institute of Obstetricians and Gynaecologists, expressing concern about the stalled project.

In my letters I expressed the Institute's support for a co-located hospital, as per international best practice, in contrast to integration, which, I wrote, 'is very far from being best practice and in fact introduces an unacceptable risk into the provision of maternity services for a variety of reasons, including adequate budget allocation, cross infection and inability to protect beds.'

In the view of the Institute, 'the NMH would be in dereliction of its responsibilities if it acquiesced to the transfer of governance of the hospital to a general hospital board which has no experience or competence whatsoever in the provision of maternity services.'

I raised St Vincent's urgent need to increase its private hospital's theatre capacity ('This should not come on the back of a new maternity hospital'), and I outlined the difficulties experienced by Cork University Maternity Hospital, where its integration with the general hospital, CUH, had resulted in the cutting of maternity, gynaecology and neonatal budgets, to the detriment of patient services. In early 2016 there were more than 4,000 women waiting for gynaecology outpatient appointments, and a gynaecology operating theatre had lain idle for almost a decade. While of course babies were delivered, treatment for women with conditions causing them misery in their daily lives – conditions such as painful heavy periods, prolapse, incontinence – was at the front line of cuts in Cork.*

---

* Though it has been gradual, as a result of continual pressure from its obstetricians and other staff, CUMH management has got increased executive and budgetary authority, and there has been considerable progress with its waiting lists. In late 2018 Professor John Higgins, recently appointed clinical director of

I also pointed out that the mastership model of leadership in maternity hospitals had been endorsed in the National Maternity Strategy, launched in January.

In my letters to the Minister for Health and the HSE, I reminded them who owned the hospital – the Religious Sisters of Charity – and the global prohibition by the Catholic Church on key gynaecological and obstetric services, drawing attention to the implications for the operation of the Protection of Life During Pregnancy Act. In my letter to the Minister, I referenced the transfer of land to the Vatican by the Sisters of Mercy in Cork and wondered:

whether or not the same process is under way with the Sisters of Charity in respect of the Elm Park site. That might perhaps be an explanation for the seemingly inexplicable rebuff by the board of SVHG on two separate occasions in recent months when you intervened personally to advance the process. It might also explain the SVHG insistence on keeping the Elm Park site unencumbered by the presence of a co-located but separately owned hospital.

I find it unacceptable that at this stage in our Republic the ownership of some of our leading, and State-funded, teaching hospitals is being secretly transferred out of the reach of the State to be vested in the Vatican. The situation now appears to be having a direct and malign influence on Irish women's reproductive health.

I put exactly the same points to James Menton in my letter to him. No response was ever forthcoming from the Department of Health and the HSE, and, indeed, a year later the Department claimed to have no knowledge of my letter. Rhona Mahony forwarded the letter I wrote to her to both the Department and the HSE.

On 11 April she wrote to me expressing her gratitude to the Institute 'for providing an opinion regarding optimum governance and control' of the new hospital. However, somewhat to my surprise, she

---

maternity services for CUMH, was able to say that, since increasing staffing, increasing the number of clinics and the numbers attending clinics, running clinics at night-time and organizing patients into groups with the same complaints, waiting lists had been substantially reduced, and that by 2019 he expected to no longer have a gynaecology waiting list. However, at the time of writing, the theatre has still not been commissioned.

told me she was unhappy that I had raised concerns about religious ethos. She wanted, she said, to confine the argument to governance only.

My view was that a row about corporate and clinical governance between two voluntary hospitals was unlikely to elicit public or political interest, whereas genuine and well-founded concerns about the influence of Catholic ethos on the medical care of women would be more successful in galvanizing opinion in favour of independent co-location.

On 1 April James Menton replied to me, denying that SVHG had proposed a full integration of hospital operations. 'Rather,' he stated, 'we have proposed a structure to enable efficient, independent hospital operations under a single system of corporate and clinical governance.' SVHG had proposed that 'NMH operations would be controlled by a clinical director and chief executive for that hospital', replacing the master, although 'matters arising from proposed changes in job descriptions can certainly be discussed and resolved. Indeed we have several years to address those issues before the relocation takes place.'

The NMH budget would be 'entirely protected by a separate service agreement with the HSE, and the maternity infrastructure would be protected by a grant agreement with the HSE. Therefore, beds, theatres, staffing, operations and funding would all be protected for the NMH.'

He stated that SVHG hospitals 'are operated in line with Irish law' and that the Protection of Life During Pregnancy Act would 'operate normally' in the NMH following the relocation. He added that '[T]he operations of NMH, and indeed SVUH, would in no way be affected by our private hospital, which is already at an advanced stage in its plans to increase its theatre and laboratory capacity. Our private and public hospitals operate independently.' At the time of going to press I am unaware of any construction at St Vincent's private hospital to increase theatre and laboratory capacity.

In my view, this response, with its generic reiteration of corporate and clinical governance practices, left unanswered the very real concerns around Catholic ethos, and in a second letter, on 18 April, I asked for clarification for the benefit of the Institute. I had by this time obtained a copy of the 'SVHG Proposed Group Structure' put to the NMH, and the full extent of what St Vincent's intended to do with the NMH was now clear.

SVHG was insisting on a reporting structure that downgraded the NMH to a division of SVHG, reporting to the SVHG board of directors, which in turn reports to the shareholders (i.e. the Sisters of Charity). An NMH oversight committee would be a subcommittee of the SVHG board, with its terms of reference set annually and its chair appointed by SVHG. This subcommittee of the board would have a three to two majority of voting members in favour of SVHG. The master would only attend this committee by invitation, and he or she would report to both a CEO of the NMH and a group clinical director of SVHG, who would in turn report to the group CEO, who would in turn report to the SVHG board of directors. I put it to Menton that, as he himself had said the shareholders – the Sisters of Charity – 'control the SVHG Board, [i]t is hard to view this structure as anything other than full integration'.

A brief letter came in response in which Menton asserted that '[T]his relocation process was instigated in order to provide women with a more closely integrated care and risk management framework that would reduce the risks presented to them in the existing system.' He cited again the need for a 'single system of clinical and corporate governance'. He finished by asserting that '[W]e have a contract with the State to provide medical services in accordance with the law. This is not affected by the views of our shareholders, and to suggest otherwise is simply incorrect.'

This statement was completely at variance with the reality for consultants working in St Vincent's. For example, neither tubal ligation nor vasectomy was permitted in the hospital. Any GP who naively wrote to St Vincent's department of gynaecology requesting a woman be considered for tubal ligation was instructed to refer that woman on to the National Maternity Hospital. The Sisters of Charity 'Health Service Philosophy and Ethical Code' of April 2010 could not be more clear:

Direct abortion is never permitted since it constitutes the intentional killing of the unborn. Also any procedures, the direct purpose of which is to destroy the embryo at any stage of its development, either by preventing it from implantation, or removing it from the womb before it is viable, or by any other procedure is not permitted . . . Direct sterilisation of either men or women is not permitted in our healthcare services when its sole immediate objective is to prevent or eliminate fertility . . . Extracorporeal conception as it is attained, for example in the process of in-vitro fertilization, bypasses the marital act and is not permissible in our healthcare services.

St Vincent's provided and continues today to provide medical services according to this ethical code. I simply could not understand James Menton's assertion to the contrary.

Meanwhile, on 1 April 2016, Rhona Mahony hosted a meeting at the NMH of an interested group of mostly women, asking for help to counter SVHG demands for integration. Orla O'Connor, the CEO of the National Women's Council of Ireland (NWCI), was in attendance, together with a good sprinkling of clinical colleagues. Journalist Dearbhail McDonald opened the meeting by summarizing the concerns in relation to the takeover of the NMH by a Catholic hospital. The master spoke next about her fears of religious interference in the new NMH. Then the meeting was opened to the floor. Towards the end a questioner asked what it would take for public opinion to be 'galvanized' on the issue. It proved a difficult question to answer.

Later in the month the master and the deputy chairman, Niall Doyle, met with Tom Lynch, chairman of the Ireland East Hospital Group (which includes St Vincent's and St Michael's among its hospitals), and Mary Day, chief executive of Ireland East, to seek their help in resolving the deadlock with St Vincent's. One solution mooted was the possible location of the NMH at the Mater Hospital. The Mater team made it clear, however, that their Catholic ethos was a barrier to any such proposal. Tom Lynch would later tell the *Sunday Times* that 'it was unanimously agreed that the co-location of NMH with St Vincent's represents the best outcome and the meeting resulted in the resolution that the IEHG would lend every assistance to bring that to fruition.'

It appeared that the NMH was now out of options for a new site. It was equally obvious that each time St Vincent's disengaged from the process, their re-engagement resulted in Holles Street ceding more ground.

★

Against this background there was a change of government. The late-February general election had not produced a decisive result, and it was not until the first week of May that a Fine Gael-led minority government took office. So, all through April I was conscious that Leo Varadkar, who favoured co-location and was on Holles Street's side in the dispute, was likely to leave the Department of Health. His successor might well take a different position.

After considerable reflection, and for the first time in my life, I decided to put a story into the public domain. I contacted Justine McCarthy of the *Sunday Times*, a rigorous journalist of great integrity with a notable body of work on important social issues. It was a serious step, although, as it turned out, I was not the only Holles Street person to brief the press in the third week of April 2016.

On 24 April the *Sunday Times* carried a front-page story with the headline 'Nuns Obstruct Maternity Hospital Plan'. Justine McCarthy had done extensive research and had contacted SVHG, the NMH and the archbishop of Dublin. She wrote that '[T]he planned relocation of the National Maternity Hospital to Elm Park in Dublin has been delayed because the SVHG, which is owned by the Religious Sisters of Charity, is insisting that it take over corporate governance. SVHG will not let completed architects' plans for the new 33,000 sq. m. institution be submitted for planning until the [NMH] agrees to become a branch of its corporate structure.'

A spokesman for the NMH told McCarthy that the hospital 'has no objection to campus management in Elm Park, but will not surrender its corporate independence', as this would end the mastership system and thereby create 'unacceptable clinical risk'. By tradition the Catholic archbishop of Dublin is the inactive chairman of the NMH. A spokeswoman for Diarmuid Martin, the current archbishop, said: 'He is aware of the difficulties but it is a matter for the boards of both hospitals to resolve.'

SVHG told McCarthy that its agreement to accommodate the NMH on its campus 'was always predicated' on the 2008 KPMG review, and warned that 'the project cannot proceed if the parties cannot agree a [single] system to follow consistent high standards for all patients on the campus.' (In fact KPMG repeatedly recommended co-location throughout the report.) The NMH countered that '[A]ll parties explicitly agreed that the 2008 KPMG report is superseded by other reports and by the current national maternity strategy', adding that 'in November 2014, SVHG set out new governance require-ments for this project to succeed, which run counter to the national maternity strategy and best practice in maternity and neonatal care.' Looking on, I could not understand how the NMH had missed a golden opportunity in the negotiations, i.e., to capitalize on the key finding of the KPMG report, which recommended co-location. The gulf between both sides was clear, and McCarthy noted that the St Vincent's board would meet the following Thursday to discuss the deadlock.

In its editorial the *Sunday Times* acknowledged the dangers I had highlighted. Under the headline 'Sisters' Power Grab is a Danger to the State', the paper argued that 'the Religious Sisters of Charity must not be allowed to get away with their audacious attempt to take control of the State's maternity services. The potential risks this power grab presents to the health of women and girls are too serious to allow for any complacency by the incoming government . . . Not only does the SVHG's stance fly in the face of the Government's national maternity strategy, it raises the spectre of a Catholic ethos determining the obstetric and gynaecological care of Ireland's female population.'

The editorial also referenced the 2013 declaration by Kevin Doran, then a priest on the Mater Hospital's board of governors, that because of its Catholic ethos the hospital could not comply with the Protec-tion of Life During Pregnancy Bill.

I had had a well-publicized spat with Fr Doran at the time, during which I had said that the Church needed to back off and leave medi-cine to the doctors. 'It is absolutely intolerable that a hospital would deny someone life-saving treatment in the twenty-first century.' At the next board meeting at the Mater, the deputy chair, my late father-in-law, Don Mahony, had asked every member to state whether or not they would implement 'the law of the land'. All members apart from Fr Doran and one of the Sisters of Mercy on the board, Sr Eugene Nolan, confirmed they would. Fr Doran left the board that October. He was appointed a bishop seven months later by Pope Francis.

On the same day as Justine McCarthy's article, Dearbhail McDon-ald, in the *Sunday Independent*, reported on the deadlock. She had been told by the NMH that St Vincent's demands would 'place all services, including tertiary maternity services at NMH, under the complete control of the St Vincent's board and shareholders, the Religious Sisters of Charity'. The NMH told McDonald that 'the elimination of the National Maternity Hospital as an entity, and the eliminating of decision-making capacity at senior clinical and corporate level, create an unacceptable clinical risk.'

SVHG responded that the question of campus governance was the 'only disagreement of significance', and that the hospital's own medical services were in accordance with the law and 'not affected by the views of our shareholders'. Once again St Vincent's were insisting that its medical services were unaffected by the ethical code of the Sisters of Charity, which was contrary to reality.

I wrote a letter on behalf of the Institute to the papers on 26 April in which I reiterated all the arguments in favour of co-location and independence, noting that the National Maternity Strategy had been developed in response to adverse incidents in maternity services in recent years. I concluded by urging the Minister, the Department of Health and the HSE to ensure that 'the National Maternity Strategy is not holed below the waterline before it has a chance to get under way'.

Chris Fitzpatrick, former master of the Coombe and the HSE representative on the project, also expressed support for the NMH, telling the *Irish Times* that Holles Street must retain its board 'in the interest of patient safety'. He noted the increasing ethical considerations 'in relation to complex issues in pregnancy', and these, he said, needed to be taken into account by those with 'long experience in maternity services'.

St Vincent's responded, publicly describing concerns over ethos as 'ridiculous', 'groundless' and 'sensationalist'. Following an SVHG board meeting in late April, James Menton wrote to the Department of Health to say that the offer to house the NMH on its Elm Park campus 'remains open for the time being', but his board saw it as 'pointless and futile in the present circumstances to engage in meetings on detailed project planning'.

He added that his board was 'extremely offended' by the NMH's 'damaging' and 'untrue' statements to the media. In response, the Department issued a statement putting its preference for the NMH's independence on the record for the first time, stating that '[C]urrent government policy is to co-locate the NMH on [the SVHG] campus, with each hospital retaining its own identity . . . and retaining the mastership model for the NMH.'

In a *Sunday Times* report Justine McCarthy noted that SVHG was 'not without support'. She had been told by Tom Lynch that 'I think their offer is a pretty fair one. It seems to meet every requirement Holles Street would have . . . All Vincent's are saying is that there should be one corporate structure but operational, budgetary and clinical independence.'

On the same day James Menton and SVHG CEO Michael Keane gave an interview to Susan Mitchell of the *Sunday Business Post* in which Menton accused the NMH of trying to string along SVHG and embarrass it into signing the letter seeking planning permission. He said that suggestions that the Sisters of Charity were trying to seize and control the maternity hospital were 'inaccurate and the cheapest shot I have seen in a long time'.

It was Professor Keane's comments, however, that brought the NMH's concerns into extremely sharp focus. It made no sense, he argued, to have integrated buildings and completely separate ownership and governance: 'This new building will have wards from St Vincent's situated in it. The theatres are going to be joined up all on one floor.' This was precisely what the NMH feared: that St Vincent's would take over some of the operating theatres, since they would all be on the same corridor. As Professor Keane described it, the new NMH would be just an extension of St Vincent's.

Just at the point where there was considerable media focus on the dispute between Holles Street and St Vincent's, and the NMH might have been expected to regain some ground, the NMH appeared to shift position. This shift can be traced to changing personnel on the NMH board. The previous December High Court president Nicholas Kearns had retired four months earlier than planned. Through the master Kearns let it be known that he wished to devote part of his retirement time to Holles Street. A small selection committee co-opted him as a governor in January 2016. As a governor he joined a body of up to 100 people who own the NMH in trust and oversee its management. The actual day-to-day management lies in the hands of the master, who reports to the twenty-one-member executive committee (board). Kearns made it clear that his condition for joining the board was that he would be appointed to the position of deputy chairman at the first available moment, which would be at the AGM towards the end of May. The current incumbent, Niall Doyle, indicated he was happy to step down. Effectively Kearns would then be the chair of the board, given the tradition that the occupant of the position of chair, the archbishop of Dublin, does not participate in board meetings. Even before the AGM Kearns became an active spokesperson on behalf of the hospital.

It was perplexing to me why Nicholas Kearns had wanted to retire early from such a prestigious position as president of the High Court and a de facto Supreme Court judge, to come to Holles Street as deputy chairman. As a matter of good governance, I and one other board member felt that he should spend at least a year, if not more, on the board prior to becoming chair. I felt it was not in the best interests of the hospital to have somebody come on to the board and become chair within a matter of months. I was particularly concerned in the case of someone who had no medical knowledge or experience of healthcare, and who had been in a position where his authority had effectively been unquestioned, given his senior position as a High Court judge for many years. My opinion remains the same. Our view did not prevail.

Kearns expressed his desire to work closely with the master in moving the project forward, offering to lead new negotiations with St Vincent's.

The NMH executive had met on 27 April to discuss a proposed third round of mediation. Once again St Vincent's had rejected the NMH nominee, and this time proposed Kieran Mulvey to mediate negotiations. The consensus of our meeting was that Mulvey, a former chief executive of the Labour Relations Commission, was an experienced and well-respected negotiator, and we would look as if we were just causing difficulties if we rejected him.

On Friday, 6 May, the day the new government was formed, Leo Varadkar, in his last intervention as Minister for Health, warned St Vincent's that it must resolve the row or the funding would be directed 'elsewhere'. This was his final attempt to get SVHG to shift position after two years of resistance.

However, instead of St Vincent's shifting position, it was the NMH that changed tack. The NMH negotiators had either lost their nerve or decided that continued resistance to St Vincent's demands was futile – which amounted to the same thing. A statement was issued saying that the NMH was 'keen to urgently resume conversation focused on overcoming the current differences to everyone's satisfaction so that this project can be realised'.

In the *Irish Times* James Menton was reported as welcoming the NMH's commitment to seeking a resolution to the impasse but also quoted as saying that it was difficult to reconcile the NMH's position with comments I had made, which he characterized as 'challenging the *bona fidés* of our board, our medical director, and our shareholders, when we state that all medical procedures currently undertaken at Holles Street can continue to be carried out in the relocated hospital at the Elm Park campus'. He added that it would 'help clarify matters greatly if Holles Street was to say whether Dr Boylan was reflecting the opinion of its board'.

I was, of course, reflecting the opinion of the board, and with the encouragement of the master, but at this point the NMH changed course. In the first sign that I was to be isolated, an NMH spokesman said that 'Dr Boylan did not speak for the hospital and was not involved in discussions on the relocation project.'

Some days later a spokesman for the NMH would say that the hospital 'had never raised ethical matters', the implication being that they had no concerns about Catholic ethos. This had not been the master's position publicly up to that point, and she had encouraged me in my efforts to defend the NMH's position.

Everything now changed. There was a new Minister for Health, Simon Harris, and a few days after his appointment on 6 May he visited Holles Street and described the delivery of the new hospital as a priority, commenting that 'the people of Ireland and expectant mothers and their families want the hospital built and do not want it bogged down in any row over ethos or governance.'

The Sunday papers that weekend should have given the Minister pause for thought. A front-page story in the *Sunday Business Post* was headlined: 'Catholic Ethos Restricting St Vincent's Hospital Doctors from Procedures'. Susan Mitchell reported that 'Gynaecologists and urologists at SVHG confirmed they were "not allowed" to perform procedures such as vasectomies and tubal ligations for patients who want to permanently prevent pregnancy. The doctors specifically contradicted assurances given by management at SVHG which had insisted there were no restrictions stopping its doctors from performing these procedures, observing that statements made by their employer in recent days were "misleading". One of the urologists at SVHG described how GP referral letters for vasectomies were returned with an explanation that it was "against the ethos of the hospital".'

Susan Mitchell had also received confirmation from Mater consultants that vasectomies and tubal ligations were not done there. John Thornhill, president of the Irish Society of Urology, confirmed that vasectomies were 'not allowed in hospitals in the public sector with a Catholic ethos'. Mitchell noted that there are no restrictions at the HSE hospitals of Beaumont, Connolly or St James's. She concluded that '[T]he latest revelation will be particularly embarrassing for SVHG.'

Far from being embarrassed, however, St Vincent's CEO, Professor Keane, would continue to insist to the *Irish Times* two days later that claims about ethical issues were a 'red herring' and a 'sideshow'. St Vincent's staff, he said, had fitted seventy Mirena coils the previous year, so that 'to contend that religious ethics are hanging over their heads when they are putting in coils is a bit rich.' What he omitted to point out, however, is that Mirena coils are also used for the control of heavy menstrual periods. Every gynaecologist in Ireland knows that Mirena coils are not inserted at St Vincent's for the purposes of contraception, but only when the indication is heavy periods. This, to me, had echoes of the practice of prescribing the pill as a 'cycle regulator' prior to the legalization of contraceptives in Ireland.

When I read Susan Mitchell's story, I felt there was a real opportunity for the NMH to press home its case with the new Minister. Surely no one could now deny that we had been right to fear the influence of Catholic ethos on the practice of medicine in St Vincent's – nothing of what was in the story was news to any of us, but here was proof for even the most sceptical observer.

At this precise point the NMH summary timeline recorded that a 'red line' had been reached by SVHG's demands that 'NMH agree to dissolve Charter and transfer ownership of land, building and company to SVHG on the grounds that there would be reserved powers to provide legal protection for clinical services.' The timeline then concludes with a comment indicating that the Holles Street negotiators understood the seriousness of the deadlock: 'The NMH agree to equal representation of SVHG on the Board of the New Company with appropriate external stakeholders. This is rejected by SVHG, who want control of the Board, no external stakeholder composition, and a quorum of SVHG members of the Board to reach decision.'

However, on the very day that Susan Mitchell's story appeared, the NMH issued a statement that astounded me. The NMH noted 'the commitment made by St Vincent's that no restrictions would be placed on its procedures. We totally accept their *bona fides* in this regard.' The deliberate repetition of the phrase *bona fides* made it clear that the NMH wanted to respond directly to James Menton's veiled insistence that I be removed from the scene.

To me this represented a complete pivot on two of the three issues of deep concern: ethos and clinical governance, leaving in play only corporate governance. The NMH statement had been issued in advance of a meeting the following day, Monday, 9 May, between Nicholas Kearns, representing the NMH, and James Menton for SVHG.

Minister Harris then intervened. Describing himself as 'appalled and horrified' by the conditions he witnessed on his visit to Holles Street, he said he would try to use his newness as Minister to bring momentum to the situation. 'There is a risk in an argument about governance that the real issue gets lost here, and that is the need to build a modern top-class facility for maternity services.' The Minister seemed to be missing the point: a controversy around governance may seem like a side issue, but it is the bedrock of institutions of integrity.

Meanwhile Justine McCarthy had been investigating the question of the transfer of ownership by the religious orders to Church control. The Mater confirmed what I had already heard: they were 'transferring the ownership of some of Ireland's biggest hospitals into a "canonical and civil entity" that will make the archbishop of Dublin responsible for ethical issues'. The paperwork for the transfer of the Mater, Cappagh and Temple Street hospitals into a canon law structure, known as a Public Juridic Person (PJP), was indeed 'awaiting the signature' of the archbishop.

A PJP is created with Vatican agreement to oversee the mission of a healthcare institution and ensure that it is carried out according to Catholic principles. Despite the name, the structure provides that a selected group of people govern what is effectively a trust, and they are appointed by nomination. McCarthy noted that the Mater group's tangible assets were valued at €635 million.

It had long been a source of puzzlement to me that the issue of the declining numbers of the religious in Ireland seemed to occasion no questioning as to what, or who, would replace them. The answer of course was that Catholic ethos does not disappear from Catholic institutions just because the religious are elderly, or are no more. Lay people, just as committed to Catholic teaching, replace them.

Tom Lynch, chairperson of both the Mater and the IEHG, confirmed to McCarthy that, following the establishment of the PJP, 'the existing board of the hospital will continue. There will be no change in its composition.' A source told McCarthy that the PJP would reserve responsibility 'for issues pertinent to ethics'.

Lynch and the Mater were perfectly open about the hospital's ethos. And yet we were being asked to believe that, just a few kilometres across the city, the Catholic ethos of St Vincent's had no influence whatsoever on their hospital. How on earth could this be credible?

13. Holles Street on the back foot

Once Kieran Mulvey was appointed to mediate between Holles Street and St Vincent's in late May 2016, the co-location controversy went quiet. The NMH executive board delegated responsibility to a team led by Nicholas Kearns and Rhona Mahony that kept the board informed on the tone and broad outline of the negotiations. Like most members of the board, I was in the dark about the details of progress until a tranche of documents was circulated in early October ahead of a special executive meeting to be held four days later. When I read these, I was at first perplexed, and then aghast. It was clear that the NMH team was very much on the back foot and desperately trying to get some structure in the agreement that would preserve the clinical independence and autonomy of the hospital.

In response to draft agreements by Mulvey in July and early August, the NMH responded on 25 August: 'Following detailed consideration by the Board of Governors [of the NMH] . . . we put forward . . . the matters which will require amendment in order for the Terms of Agreement to be accepted by the Governors.'

The NMH memorandum went on to say that Holles Street was willing to concede to a board of directors comprised of five SVHG appointees and four NMH directors, 'provided the "reserved powers" are exercised by the four NMH Directors only', and that the SVHG directors would not cast a vote in relation to the reserved powers. The so-called reserved powers were provisions intended to ensure clinical and operational independence.

The memorandum said that it was the 'unanimous view' of the NMH governors that 'without either (a) a majority on the board or (b) a set of reserved functions for decision exclusively by the NMH appointed directors, the clinical independence and autonomy of the hospital cannot be preserved. The Governors cannot support the proposed relocation without firm either option (a) or failing that option (b) being inserted into the terms of agreement.'

The NMH memorandum was wrong on a number of levels. First,

draft terms of agreement had never been put to the governors – or indeed to the executive. There had been no consideration of any kind by the governors. Why had the mediator been told that the governors had a unanimous view when nothing had been put to us? Second, I could not understand how the suggestion that the five SVHG directors would not be able to vote on the 'reserved powers' could ever work in real life on a board. I was both disturbed and increasingly angered.

There was worse to come. Included in the papers was a copy of a letter written by Nicholas Kearns and Rhona Mahony to Kieran Mulvey on 15 September. It was clear from reading it that in the space of three weeks further ground had been lost. Kearns and Mahony expressed their disappointment with the latest document from Kieran Mulvey, telling him that '[W]e feel strongly that the paper does not reflect our position, nor does it take account of progress made over the last few weeks.' However, it also said:

We are willing to dissolve the Charter and agree that the ownership of what is now the NMH will transfer to the ownership of SVHG, a private company owned by the Sisters of Charity. This will be effected through the creation of a new company ('New NMH'), which will be a 100 per cent owned subsidiary of SVHG. This is a major concession and requires legal protection in the interests of women and infants.

They added: '[I]n accordance with the SVHG requirements for co-location, we are willing to cede ownership of the maternity hospital building.'

Cede ownership? Dissolve the charter? But the NMH is owned in trust by its governors, who must agree on any disposal of assets. And dissolution of the NMH as a corporate entity would require the passage of an Act of the Oireachtas, as it was set up with a charter granted by King Edward VII in 1903. Yet Kearns and Mahony – in my view under pressure, and clearly without the knowledge or agreement of either the executive committee or the governors – had unilaterally offered to surrender the independence of the 122-year-old maternity hospital to a private company owned in full by an order of Catholic sisters.

This concession was breath-taking on a number of levels. Nicholas Kearns had occupied the position of deputy chairman for less than four months. And was Rhona Mahony's legacy as first female master of the National Maternity Hospital to be its surrender to the Catholic Church?

The documents showed that an intense three weeks of negotiations followed this letter as the mediation process reached the final stage. In a letter to Mahony on 6 October, Simon Harris made it clear that government patience was running out.

The following day the master replied to the Minister that she remained concerned that

the mediator has been unable to achieve the appointment of an independent director. The proposal that the independent director should be the UCD nominee who currently sits on the SVHG board does not fulfil the criteria of independence, and independent legal opinion obtained by the hospital confirms this unequivocally.

She concluded her letter by assuring the Minister that, '[w]hile I will continue to do all I can to contribute to bring this process to a successful outcome, I must advise you that this will ultimately be an independent board decision. The hospital has scheduled an extraordinary general meeting so that the board can make its decision on the proposal put to the hospital.'

But an EGM had *not* been scheduled: the forthcoming meeting was a special meeting of the executive only.

Furthermore, it was clear that the master and deputy chairman, in the letter of 15 September, had already conceded the substantive issues and, as far as I could see, were pushing back on one issue alone: the independence or otherwise of the ninth member of the board. To my mind, this was rearranging the deckchairs on the *Titanic*. Independence had always been the key objective, but, having already conceded full control and ownership to SVHG, this last stand seemed too little, too late.

As the negotiations came to a conclusion in October 2016, there were difficult discussions about the composition of the board. The only concession the NMH could wring from the process was that the ninth director 'shall be an independent international expert in Obstetrics and Gynaecology' and not the UCD 'Group Academic Nominee' who already sat on the board of SVHG. Crucially, however, the ninth director would be appointed by a selection committee of three, chaired by the SVHG clinical director, and with the SVHG CEO and a representative from the NMH – i.e., a built-in SVHG majority. So much for independence.

When the executive met on the evening of Tuesday, 11 October, in the boardroom at Holles Street, the proposition put before us was indeed characterized as the deal presented, or no deal at all. The mood at the meeting was tense. I raised my concerns, again, on the three key issues: ownership and control, governance and the potential for the interference of Catholic ethos.

Any attempt to raise the issue of the influence of Catholic ethos was vociferously rejected by the master. It was claimed that the 'reserved powers' would safeguard the NMH's interests, but I remained unconvinced by that on the evidence in front of me.

A vote was taken. Four members present did not back the proposed relocation agreement: all three of the previous masters, i.e., myself, Declan Keane and Mike Robson (who between us had run the hospital for twenty-one years), together with the solicitor Kevin Mays, who had been a governor of the hospital since 1992. In fact I abstained in the vote out of loyalty to Rhona Mahony, who is my wife's sister. It was a gesture in what was a difficult family situation; as the voting was clearly overwhelmingly in favour, another vote against wasn't going to make any difference. A fifth member who could not attend, Councillor Mícheál Mac Donncha, had written to the board's secretary in advance, noting that the NMH had already made very significant concessions and that St Vincent's insistence on effective control of the new board therefore seemed 'entirely unreasonable'.

The rest of the board, however, were persuaded that they had to accept what the master and deputy chairman had already agreed. I counted several recent appointees to the executive around the table, individuals who had no medical background, and was astounded, given that none of the three previous masters could support the proposal, that they were happy to sign off on the draft agreement. I could discern no evidence that they had made any attempt to acquaint themselves with canon law and with how Catholic hospitals around the world are run. They had been appointed to the board because of their expertise in the fields of law, accounting, stockbroking and other professions, but they seemed to have ignored the most basic principles of due diligence. Nor did it seem that the mediator had even considered the question of canon law and the ownership structure of the new hospital. It seemed that a boiler-plate Irish mediation solution had been imposed. The best I felt I could do that evening was to secure an undertaking from the deputy chairman that no final decisions or agreements would be made until the proposal was put to the governors at an EGM. As this book goes to press more than three years later, it has still not been put to the NMH governors.

Kieran Mulvey's report was presented to Minister Harris on 21 November. It was immediately apparent that there had been two significant changes to the document put to the NMH executive five weeks earlier, amendments that had not been communicated to us.

Mulvey told the Minister in Section B (1) [Establishment of New Company] that 'A Designated Activity Company (DAC), *limited by shares*, to be established under the Companies Act 2014 (reference *Part 16* Companies Act 2014). *This DAC will be a 100% subsidiary of SVHG* and which [*sic*] will allow for an objects clause and facilitate charitable status [my italics].'

However, what the NMH executive had endorsed in the draft report put to us in the 11 October special meeting was section B (1) which read simply 'A new Company to be established under the Companies Act 2014. (*Company Limited by Guarantee – Part 18* of the Act.)' The draft report on which we had voted had stated that the new company was to be owned solely by SVHG, but nowhere was there any reference to the NMH being a '100% subsidiary of SVHG'. (Although in their letter of 15 September to the mediator, Nicholas Kearns and Rhona Mahony had written that the 'New NMH' would be 'a 100 per cent owned subsidiary of SVHG').

Under this configuration, the so-called 'reserved powers' were completely meaningless as protection for the NMH's independence. What on earth had happened?

There was no attempt in the Mulvey Report to address the issue of Catholic ethos. When I continued to raise concerns about religious interference, I was pointed to the reserved power which provided for 'the provision of maternity, gynaecological, obstetrics and neonatal services without religious, ethnic or other distinction'. This of course referred to the religious or ethnic background of the *patients*, not the nature of the care that would be made available to them. This line would be repeatedly trotted out over the coming months.

It was immensely frustrating.

I had more questions as I read through the report.

Would either side have a majority on the board?

Yes, SVHG would.

Would the ninth director be the chair of the board of the new NMH?

No. The chair would rotate every three years between nominees of the NMH and SVHG. I simply could not understand why someone from SVHG should be chair of the board of the National Maternity Hospital.

How had the negotiating team done in preserving the NMH's clinical independence?

It was claimed that the mastership model as outlined in the National Maternity Strategy would be retained, but, according to the 'Clinical Governance Structure' outlined in the Mulvey Report, the master would in fact be one of four clinical directors and well down the organizational hierarchy. These doctors would report to both the group clinical director and the group medical board medical executive, who in turn would report to the group CEO, who would in turn continue to report to the SVHG board of directors, who, as we knew, answered to the Sisters of Charity. (Tellingly, this structure was practically identical to the one set out in the document 'SVHG Proposed Group Structure' that it had presented to the NMH prior to Kieran Mulvey's involvement in the negotiations; St Vincent's hadn't budged an inch.) There was no role for the new NMH Designated Activity Company anywhere in this structure. So would the NMH DAC maybe have a role in campus governance?

No, it would not.

Finally, the report gave the Minister for Health a 'Golden Share' in the hospital, an apparent veto over any action of the board that would not protect the reserved powers, that might jeopardize the state's investment or be out of line with government policy. So, did this Golden Share have any legal standing?

No, it did not (and still doesn't, because no legal agreement has been drawn up). Ludicrously, it could be exercised only when there was unanimity on the board – in other words a mechanism to solve a dispute required the board to all vote together.

I could only conclude that the NMH negotiators had been out-
manoeuvred by SVHG, and not helped by the mediator. It was also
my strong impression that there was a desperate desire to get a new
hospital built, or at least for building to commence, within Rhona
Mahony's tenure, and that this desire was shared by the new deputy
chairman, Nicholas Kearns.

The Mulvey Report had not yet been put to the NMH governors
when, the day after the executive meeting on 23 November, during
which I again strongly expressed my concerns, the Department of
Health issued a press statement in which the Minister declared himself 'thrilled to be in a position today to launch the development of
this vital project'. He thanked Kieran Mulvey for putting the agreement together, describing it as 'fair, balanced and workable', and said
that 'the move to the Elm Park campus will ensure the continuation
of the ethos and tradition of the National Maternity Hospital, in a
modern environment which meets best international standards.'

Meanwhile the media concluded, as Martin Wall and Paul Cullen
put it in the *Irish Times*, that an 'unedifying spat [had] delayed an
urgently needed move from outdated city premises'. They reported
that '[T]he company will be 100 per cent owned by St Vincent's Hospital Group, but will enjoy clinical and operational independence in
the provision of maternity, gynaecology, obstetrics and gynaecology
services.' The dispute had been 'mostly over governance issues', but
they noted my concerns over Catholic ethos.

When the minutes from the November executive meeting were
circulated, they had been sanitized to the point where none of the
concerns I had raised were recorded. At my insistence, the minutes
were revised to read:

The Deputy Chair advised that the Governors would need to approve the
final document. Dr Peter Boylan expressed his reservations including that the
DAC would be a 100 per cent subsidiary of SVUH (Sisters of Charity) and
that we were effectively transferring ownership of NMH to SVUH and
improving the SVUH balance sheet by €150 million. He also noted his concerns on the operation of the Selection Committee [for the ninth director] in
spite of veto . . . He expressed concern about the bona fides of SVUH and
that the 'seamless provision of care' would be used as an excuse to take over
NMH facilities. Overall he continued to be concerned regarding SVUH.

Mike Robson asked for the following to be inserted: 'Dr Robson noted that he had similar concerns to Dr Boylan, but in particular in relation to the clinical governance and accountability structure.'

The Mulvey agreement was not a legally binding document. Nor, at the time of writing, has any such legal document been finalized, and the governors of the National Maternity Hospital have yet to be asked to vote on such a document, as was promised by the deputy chairman on repeated occasions.

I retired from clinical work at the National Maternity Hospital on 31 December 2016 but remained on the executive and as a governor of the hospital. At each executive meeting in the early months of 2017, I pressed for confirmation of a date for the promised EGM of the governors to discuss the Mulvey Report. It became increasingly clear that there was little interest in such a meeting from the majority of the executive members, and that Mulvey was, in effect, a *fait accompli*.

In the spring of 2017 two shocking stories, placing the religious orders directly under the news spotlight, came to light in Ireland.

On 3 March the Commission of Investigation into Mother and Baby Homes chaired by Judge Yvonne Murphy announced that 'significant' quantities of human remains, aged between thirty-five fetal weeks and two to three years, had been found in Tuam during a test excavation in a large sewage system under the site of a home run between 1925 and 1961 by the Bon Secours order.

Research published some years earlier by the local historian Catherine Corless had established that over these years some 796 death certificates had been issued for infants and young children with no indication as to burial place. Now it seemed clear that many of these children had been interred in what was described as a septic tank. There was widespread public shock and revulsion, and Taoiseach Enda Kenny made a powerful statement in the Dáil expressing a sense of national shame that women and children were treated so harshly in Ireland's past.

Then, on 9 March, the Minister for Education, Richard Bruton, spoke in a debate in the Seanad on the state Residential Institutions Redress Board (RIRB), which had been set up in 2002 to compensate victims of abuse in residential institutions run by the religious orders in the twentieth century. In 2009 the Commission to Inquire into Child Abuse chaired by Judge Sean Ryan established that neglect and physical, sexual and emotional abuse had been endemic and systematic in orphanages, industrial schools and reformatories for children over a 35-year period, identifying 800 abusers in 200 institutions. At the time the *Irish Times* had described the devastating report as 'a map of Irish hell . . . a land of pain and shame, of savage cruelty and callous indifference'.

Minister Bruton told the Seanad that over €1.5 billion had been paid in compensation by the state, and although it had been envisaged that the state and religious orders would contribute 50–50, the religious at that point had contributed only €209 million, or just over 13 per cent of the total.

In the first week of April, Patsy McGarry ran a series of articles in the *Irish Times* reporting that one of the eighteen religious congregations, the Missionary Oblates of Mary Immaculate, was of the view, shared by all the congregations, that, as the state had put together the redress scheme without their input, they felt under no 'moral pressure' to pay any more, and certainly not the 50 per cent sought by the government.

I read Patsy McGarry's report while in London at a conference of the Royal College of Obstetricians and Gynaecologists. Sitting under a flowering magnolia beside the lake in nearby Regent's Park, I thought about the words of the American judge Louis D. Brandeis: 'Publicity is justly commended as a remedy for social and industrial diseases. Sunlight is said to be the best of disinfectants.'

As matters stood, the Sisters of Charity were going to be given 100 per cent ownership of the new €300 million taxpayer-funded national maternity hospital without the full implications of the Mulvey Report being grasped. It made me angry, and I believed the public, and particularly the women of Ireland, would be outraged if they understood fully just what was being proposed. It seemed to me, therefore, that seeing the story through the lens of Patsy McGarry's reports might focus opinion. So, for the second time in my life, and almost a year to the day after I got in touch with Justine McCarthy, I made the decision to talk to a journalist I trusted and respected. I phoned Patsy McGarry at the *Irish Times*.

On Tuesday, 18 April, a short piece appeared on page 7 of that newspaper: 'Nuns to Own New Maternity Hospital'. Patsy McGarry reported that the Sisters of Charity had paid only €2 million of the €5 million offered by them after the Ryan Report, and had yet to complete the transfer of the Sacred Heart Centre in Waterford to the state as promised, yet they were to be 'given ownership of the new €300 million state-funded national maternity hospital'.★

A Department of Health spokesman said that the autonomy of the NMH board would be underpinned by reserved powers to ensure clinical and operational independence and that the Minister for Health would hold the power to protect those reserved powers.

The story caught fire immediately when the next day the Magdalene Survivors Together group expressed 'deep anger and absolute shock' at the government's decision to award sole ownership of the hospital to the Sisters of Charity. Colm O'Gorman, executive director of Amnesty International, said his 'fundamental difficulty' was with the state 'gifting a €300 million hospital to a religious congregation which has yet to honour a 15-year-old commitment to redress'. The word 'gifting' immediately caught on. Opposition politicians expressed deep unhappiness with the government's proposed course of action.

Within twenty-four hours of the first story appearing in the *Irish Times*, a protest was held outside the Department of Health, and a number of protests by the Parents for Choice group had been organized for Saturday outside St Vincent's, Holles Street and hospitals in Limerick, Cork, Galway and Drogheda. A petition was started by the campaigning organization Uplift, asking the Minister for Health 'not to hand our maternity hospital over to the Sisters of Charity', with 30,000 signatures received by Thursday. A day later more than 65,000 people had signed, and two days later, on the Sunday, signatures had exceeded 80,000.

When the story had first emerged nearly a year earlier, agreement had not been reached by the two hospitals, but now the NMH/Vincent's project was more concrete and the realization was dawning publicly that a religious order – that was subject to a state commission of inquiry on how, in the twentieth century, it ran its institutions,

---

★ The estimated building cost of the new hospital had now risen to €300 million, largely as a result of building inflation.

where mothers, infants and children were abused – would now own the 21st-century, state-of-the-art national maternity hospital.

On the morning of Thursday, 20 April, the *Irish Times* carried a piece on its front page. A journalist had asked Sr Agnes Reynolds, one of the two members of the Sisters of Charity on the SVHG board, if the congregation's ownership of the new NMH would influence the medical care given to women. She declined to comment, saying '[I] can't make a judgement on that.' She added that the new hospital would 'always respect the rights of the mother and baby . . . and reach out to all creeds and backgrounds'.

To me this sounded alarmingly proprietorial. Sr Agnes was already speaking for the new NMH. Even more worrying, unlike the lay members of her board, she ducked the question of the influence of her order's Catholic ethos on the medical care of women.

Having read the story that morning, I went on to *Morning Ireland*. I said my concerns were that the Sisters of Charity would have 100 per cent ownership of the new hospital, that the sisters would be the sole owners of the company set up to run the hospital, and that the board structure was unsatisfactory. I said that the point about full independence had been exposed by Sr Agnes and her comments, and that, although she had had an opportunity to say they would not interfere in clinical decisions, she had not done so.

We were being asked to believe, I said, that the new hospital would be the 'first hospital in the world . . . run by a company which is owned by the Catholic Church to allow things like IVF, sterilization, abortion, gender-reassignment surgery etc. This would be absolutely unique in the world and it is just not credible.'

I said that, while I fully supported the current master, and recognized the need for a new hospital, in my view Dr Mahony had been 'backed into a corner by the Minister for Health, who appeared to be saying that it was either this option or it won't happen . . . It is completely unacceptable that €300 million of our money – state money – is being given to the Sisters of Charity to build a hospital.'

Less than two hours later, Rhona Mahony and Nicholas Kearns went on Sean O'Rourke's RTÉ radio show. The master said that she was 'really surprised that the chairman of the IOG would be so misleading on radio to suggest that the nuns would be running the hospital'. This misinterpretation – that the sisters would be involved in the day-to-day running of the hospital as in the days of matrons of old, rather than my substantive points about ownership and ethos – would be repeated over the coming months. Although the new NMH would be 100 per cent owned by the Sisters of Charity and a 100 per cent subsidiary of SVHG, Dr Mahony insisted that when the NMH moved to Elm Park

[it] will be an independent hospital and an independent company with its own independent board . . . The services we provide at NMH at the moment are absolutely protected under the reserved powers . . . There will not be any religious ethos. The ownership of the public hospital is not really here nor there . . . I couldn't care less who owns my hospital building but I really care that I have control over the service that I deliver and that I can give clinical care to women that is appropriate.

She insisted that a 'triple lock' – reserved powers, a 'Golden Share' and ministerial veto – would guarantee independence.

I listened with mounting dismay. The attack was personal and the tone was emotional. Rhona Mahony omitted to say that her term of office as master would end a year and a half later, on 31 December 2018, so she would have no way of guaranteeing the independence of 'her' hospital beyond that date. She called for people 'to get behind this hospital and get it built . . . What we don't need is misinformation and scaremongering and completely inaccurate information.'

Nicholas Kearns said that it was difficult to understand my position, since I was a serving member of the board of the National Maternity Hospital. He said that as a former lawyer he was satisfied with the legal agreement, which he regarded as 'watertight and sound', and that it would safeguard the NMH's independence. He added that the new hospital would operate without religious or ethnic distinction, and that 'under the reserved powers it will be clinically and operationally independent'.

There was, however, no legal agreement in place at that time. The Mulvey Report had explicitly stated in its conclusion that '[I]t will be necessary for the appropriate legal mechanisms to be put in place regarding . . . structure, objectives, role, and powers.'

As always in these things, the devil was going to be in the detail, so I could not understand how Kearns could describe as 'watertight and sound' a 'legal agreement' that did not exist. What Kieran Mulvey had submitted to the Minister for Health was a *report* that would require future legal underpinning.

As the master and Kearns spoke, my phone started beeping. The consensus among friends and colleagues, which I shared, was that they had lost an opportunity to reassure listeners. The angry tone had not been persuasive. Several wondered if it was an exercise in 'nice cop, nasty cop' that we had planned together. Not so, unfortunately. I was clearly on the other side to the master and deputy chairman.

The following day, Friday, 21 April, there was comprehensive TV, radio and newspaper coverage. The tenor of the headlines was to question the credibility of assertions that the Sisters of Charity would not control a maternity hospital located at St Vincent's and to suggest that women were right to be nervous about the plan.

I had an opinion piece in the *Irish Times* reiterating my points. I used the opportunity to emphasize three key issues. First, that no arrangement had been put to the governors of the NMH, who must agree to any deal. Second, given the proposed board structure of the new hospital, I wondered who would win in any power struggle (the owners of the hospital, I suggested). Finally, I asked, if the safeguards for clinical independence were so robust, why was there any need for the Minister to hold a 'Golden Share'? I concluded by calling on the Minister to 'intervene to protect both the medical interests of women and their infants and the financial interests of the Irish taxpayer'.

Minister Harris came out to agree that the hospital must have 'clinical, operational and financial independence, with no question of religious interference and with a role for the Minister of Health of the day to guarantee this . . . [t]he state's financial and public health interest in the hospital must be fully protected . . . Before any contracts are entered into these criteria must be satisfied in full.' When asked about my comments on *Morning Ireland*, he stated that '[T]here will be no financial gain to any religious order from the development of this hospital' and that the HSE would put in place appropriate legal mechanisms. He said that he had heard 'legitimate questions and opinions in recent days'.

St Vincent's then followed their usual course of action by threatening once more to disengage, announcing plans to review the status of the project, prompted, they said, by 'controversy and misinformation' and by the views expressed by the Minister. The project was now 'in jeopardy', they said. A subsequent editorial in the *Irish Daily Mail* called the response from St Vincent's a 'petulant act [which] will be interpreted as an attempt to blackmail the government into accepting their terms'.

There was near-blanket coverage of the issues in that weekend's media. The narrative widened to the relationship between the state and the Catholic Church in the provision of Irish healthcare services, and the deliberations of the Citizens' Assembly, which happened to be holding its final meeting that weekend.

It emerged that the agreement between the NMH and St Vincent's had not been discussed by the Cabinet prior to being announced, as, according to a government spokesman, the agreement was between two voluntary hospitals. Simon Harris attempted to play down St Vincent's criticism of his comments during the week, arguing that he had merely asked to be allowed to do his job and that '[I]t would be betraying women and infants if we don't give this issue the time and space that it required to get it absolutely legally and contractually correct.'

The Mulvey Report had not been published, and Fianna Fáil's Billy Kelleher, the party's spokesman on health, led calls for its release. Initially the Minister refused to publish the report, saying that instead he would make it available to the Oireachtas Health Committee. Not surprisingly it was leaked, causing Billy Kelleher to comment that he found it extraordinary that 'after many days of intense speculation, it now seems the agreement reached regarding the new NMH does in fact allow St Vincent's to play a role in clinical governance. This contradicts previous statements by the Minister for Health.'

The comments of Fine Gael TD Michael Darcy showed that politicians were getting it – this was not a sideshow but a fundamental issue that was at stake. He acknowledged that 'it's hit a raw nerve. People are agitated about this. I don't think it's appropriate in this era that [the hospital] is owned by the order. What I would urge is for the deal to be looked at again and a new arrangement to be put into place to make the state the owner of the facility.'

Of course, voices were raised in support of the project as it stood. Kieran Mulvey criticized 'abuse' and 'threats' directed at SVHG and called for cool heads. He was perturbed that the improvement in women's health had been 'lost in all the argument, the rhetoric . . . Any attempt to change the agreement in its essential form will put us back to the starting blocks.' The deal, he said, would stand.

Journalist Dearbhail McDonald expressed her concerns about the agreement in the *Sunday Independent* but added, 'I honestly believe that, in the circumstances, this was and is the best deal for Irish women.'

This sentiment undoubtedly reflected the NMH opinion, but that was exactly the problem: it was the best deal they could get *as far as they believed*. However, it was not going to be the best deal for Irish women. For McDonald, responding to the evident fury of Irish women in particular in the previous days, 'It would be a tragic irony if we, as women, bring the curtain down on the one thing – high-quality maternity and reproductive care – we desperately need by conflating Catholic ethos with the money trail and the realpolitik.' Rhona Mahony was quoted in the *Sunday Times* as telling a colleague that she feared that 'the feminists are going to unravel this fantastic hospital for women.'

Support for my concerns over Catholic ethos came now, however, from the Church itself. The *Sunday Times* carried a front-page story by Justine McCarthy under the headline 'Bishop Says New Hospital Must Obey the Church'. In the story Kevin Doran, the bishop of Elphin and chair of the Irish hierarchy's committee on bioethics, told McCarthy that '[a] healthcare organization bearing the name Catholic, while offering care to all who need it, has a special responsibility . . . to Catholic teachings about the value of human life and the dignity and the ultimate destiny of [the] human person. Public funding, while it brings with it other legal and moral obligations, does not change that responsibility.' He referenced the three tenets that decree that land held by religious institutions is 'ecclesiastical property' over which the pope has 'primacy of governance'.

It did not escape my notice that, unlike other occasions, not a single member of the hierarchy came forward to dispute the bishop's opinion.

In the same article Tom Lynch of the Mater and IEHG was reported as confirming to Jim Breslin, Secretary General of the Department of Health, precisely what I had said all along – that 'canon law obliges the hospital on Catholic land to operate by Catholic rules.'

It was surely crystal-clear by now – if any arm of the Catholic Church owned the land on which the new hospital was to be built, then the NMH would be subject to canon law.

This did not mean that all was lost in terms of co-locating at St Vincent's. The Sisters of Charity owned land adjacent to the hospital campus. So, for instance, could a site be provided from the Caritas Home or Elm Park Golf Club? The state could have acquired it or the sisters could have donated it. If necessary, the hospitals could then be connected by underground and over-ground corridors, as happens on shared hospital campuses around the world. Such a solution would remove the spectre of the Catholic ethos, permit the state to own the new hospital, and also give the new national maternity hospital access to the relevant specialties at St Vincent's.

Observing the widespread coverage in the Sunday papers and morning radio shows, I concluded that the pressure on the Minister for Health was not going to abate. A senior government Minister got in touch with me that Sunday morning, wanting to talk to me ahead of meetings that week, including Tuesday's Cabinet meeting, I presumed. It seemed likely that Simon Harris would have to move his position. Statements from his Department were hinting that a review of the Mulvey Report was inevitable.

As with the previous May, here was a perfect opportunity for the NMH to row back on the hasty and over-egged defence of the deal to date, surf the wave of public and opposition political opinion, and win concessions on governance and control.

Over the course of that weekend I had noted that many papers reproduced photographs of Rhona Mahony and Simon Harris side by side, with a model of the proposed new NMH when the planning application was submitted the previous month. As political pressure mounted, I was concerned that Rhona might be caught in a damaging slipstream.

Not only is Rhona my sister-in-law but I knew her as a junior colleague for ten years before her sister Jane and I met and married, and I had vigorously supported her election as master, as I believed she had the qualities to be an effective master; I also thought it would lend great prestige to the NMH to have the first female master. I am twenty years older than her and, naturally, we have different personalities and approaches to life, but we are closely linked by family. I know how stressful the controversy was for my parents-in-law, in particular, and so I thought it was about time that Rhona and I should pull together and try to work with each other towards a better outcome for Holles Street.

Nicholas Kearns, meanwhile, I have known for more than fifty years. Nicky, as he is generally known, was a few years ahead of me in school at St Mary's College in Rathmines, and we have many mutual friends. As is the way of Dublin, our paths crossed professionally and personally for many years. Knowing both Nicky and Rhona so well, I knew they would be smarting from the negative media coverage.

After the Sunday lunchtime radio news covering the story finished on 23 April, I sent them a joint text:

> I'm sorry it has come to this but I did try to warn you. The way out for both of you is to make it clear that you were misled by SVHG, you accepted their bona fides and assurances. Both of you and the Minister are inextricably linked and you will either sink or swim together. The way to get the hospital is to insist on CPO of Elm Park golf club land on the periphery and establish links to SVH via tunnels/corridors. Minimal design alterations needed. Peter

Three hours later, I got a text back which read:

> Both the master and I have received your text sent to us at 13.47 today. We are now asking for your immediate resignation from the board of Holles St – both because of your public intervention to criticise the overwhelming majority decision of the board taken in November last to approve the agreement reached with SVUH for the transfer of Holles St to Elm Park – a vote on which you abstained – and in addition because of the content of your text sent today. Its intimidatory tone is most regrettable. The board will clearly require to be briefed on Wednesday as to the content of your text communication if your resignation as sought is not forthcoming.

I did not reply to the text. With the benefit of hindsight, I can see that the tone of my text, while not intimidatory, was not conciliatory, which I regret. It expressed the frustration and fear I was feeling about the future of the hospital.

Clearly, we were not going to work together, and it appeared that the master and the deputy chair remained wedded to the deal, in spite of the public furore. I decided I would say nothing until the board meeting, which would be taking place three days later, on Wednesday,

26 April. However, on Monday afternoon I got a phone call from Paul Cullen of the *Irish Times*. The demand for my resignation had been leaked to him. Clearly, pressure was going to be applied through the media before the board meeting.

The *Irish Times* ran a front-page story on Tuesday, quoting an NMH spokesman who confirmed that Kearns had asked me to resign from the board, adding, 'Last week, some five months after the agreement was approved, Boylan, without warning, consultation with, or notification to the board, its chair or the master of the hospital, went public in attacking the agreement. Board members have a duty of loyalty to the board on which they serve and for this reason his resignation has been sought.'

My feeling is that board members have a duty to the patients served by the hospital, and that this duty supersedes unquestioning duty to the board itself. Paul Cullen added that it was 'understood the decision to seek Dr Boylan's resignation was taken following consultation with board members, who were said to be overwhelmingly supportive'.

This statement came as a surprise to many members of the board, some of whom called me to say that they had been told nothing before reading about it in the paper.

I commented to Eilis O'Regan in the *Irish Independent* that '[I]t is shooting the messenger to ask me to resign. Telling me "you are out" is not going to advance the hospital . . . it is important to have a board with diverse opinions.'

Away from what I perceived as the bunker mentality at the NMH, the political weather was changing. In a poll on *Claire Byrne Live* on the Monday evening, a majority of 86 per cent had said the Catholic Church should have no role in maternity services, and just 7 per cent thought they should.

It was reported that the bishop of Elphin's comments had caused disquiet within government. In his *Irish Examiner* column, former government adviser Fergus Finlay wrote, 'After days of reassurance that the hospital would operate on the basis of an ethos that owed nothing to any religion, its owners (if they are its owners) are told by a bishop that this isn't the case at all. This is crazy and it gets crazier by the day . . . If the Dáil is not in uproar this week, demanding to see the agreement on which all this is based, it won't be doing its job.

It is unconscionable, and utterly unacceptable, that a vital matter of public policy, and a huge public investment, should be undertaken on the basis of a secret deal . . . The state wouldn't build a university, or any higher institute of education, and hand it over to a religious order.'

In a statement St Vincent's once again said that 'in line with current policy and procedures at SVHG, any medical procedure which is in accordance with the laws of the Republic of Ireland will be carried out in the new hospital.' But repeating the same statement over and over doesn't make it true. According to the statement, after my interview on *Morning Ireland*, the board felt 'compelled to respond to the continued misinformation and untruthful allegations being made by him concerning the medical care which will be available to women attending the new hospital'. According to the *Irish Times*, '[S]ources say the more conciliatory approach by St Vincent's followed the call by the NMH deputy chairman, Nicholas Kearns, for its former master Peter Boylan to resign.'

Declan Keane was interviewed on Tuesday's *Six One News*. Clearly uncomfortable, he expressed respect for me 'as a clinician and a colleague. But when he goes against the consensus of the NMH I can see the difficult position he put the chairman in.' He did not mention that he had voted against the proposed deal the previous October.

On *Prime Time* later that evening Rhona Mahony insisted that she and the deputy chairman were not trying to silence me. 'Not at all, it's simply a matter of corporate governance, and that's for the chairman and the rest of the board. The deal absolutely guarantees operational independence.'

On the other hand, Chris Fitzpatrick, a former master of the Coombe, who was on the HSE project board for the new hospital, had written to the HSE to say that '[I]t is wholly inappropriate in 21st-century pluralist Ireland that the ownership of this publicly funded women and infant's hospital should be entrusted in any way, shape or form to a religious organization of any denomination.' One of the Dublin City Council's two NMH board members, Councillor Mícheál Mac Donncha, told the *Irish Daily Mail* that '[T]he idea that Peter Boylan should be asked to resign because of his public comments – that is totally unacceptable . . . The majority of the board were influenced very much by the master of the hospital, Rhona Mahony, who is very well respected, very well qualified, and by Nicholas Kearns, who, with Rhona Mahony, negotiated the agreement, and we were very swayed by them, very influenced by them, that the agreement reached was a safeguard of the clinical independence of the hospital.'

Significantly, media reports had it that 'the Government believes the ownership structure of the new hospital will have to be changed in response to public concern. [Harris] will ask the boards of the two institutions to enter a month-long process in a bid to agree a new ownership structure.' Here now, it seemed, was the opportunity for Holles Street to get a better deal than the Mulvey agreement.

14. The saddest day of my career

The morning of the board meeting the *Irish Times* reported that Rhona Mahony, Declan Keane and twenty-five other Holles Street consultants had signed a letter endorsing the relocation plan. 'We believe this move must take place as urgently as possible for the sake of the women and infants we serve. The clinical arguments must not be derailed by misleading sensationalism.' The report continued that 'although not every consultant has so far signed the letter, Dr Boylan is understood to be the only consultant who has refused to sign it.'

As I had retired four months earlier, I was no longer on the consultant staff, so that was simply nonsense. Calls and texts followed immediately from colleagues who had not signed the letter or had signed it under what they felt was duress, angry at the misrepresentation. The circulation of the letter and release of the story was clearly engineered to shore up support for the Mulvey Report prior to the crucial board meeting. Given the number of non-medics on the board, that so many doctors favoured it might carry some weight.

I arrived for the board meeting shortly before 5 p.m. I looked forward to discussing the issues with the full executive board. However, the four-hour meeting was a most uncomfortable one. While some board members were sympathetic, I could feel hostility emanating from others and I made no ground in presenting my arguments.

It did not seem to me that those present had made any effort to inform themselves of canon law and Catholic teaching on reproductive healthcare. More than a year before, I had asked for just one example of a hospital anywhere in the world built on land owned by a Catholic organization that performed sterilization or abortion. Unsurprisingly, I was still waiting for an answer, as there was no such example.

Nothing I said could sway opinion. The master and the deputy chair were adamant that it was this deal or no deal, and that they were absolutely confident that none of the concerns I had raised were valid. Most of the board seemed utterly disconnected from the controversy raging outside the boardroom. The Labour councillor Brendan Carr summed up the mood for the *Irish Daily Mail*:

Peter Boylan got a very hostile reception. He didn't seem to have the support of many people in the room. There was a clear attempt to dismiss everything he said and he obviously felt himself that he could no longer contribute to that board . . . I, through my job [as a trade unionist], have dealt with a lot of hostile employers . . . but I've never witnessed anything like I witnessed at that board meeting. The hostility towards a few people of the board who tried to raise concerns from the public was absolutely disgraceful and shocking . . . This is a clear case of, if you don't do as we say, you're not welcome here.

I was not asked to resign that evening. Nor did I resign. A vote, however, was taken re-endorsing the Mulvey Report. Only Brendan Carr, Mícheál Mac Donncha and I voted against it.

The following morning Rhona Mahony said on *Newstalk Breakfast* that '[N]o misinformation or sideshow must get in the way of this focus . . . [The hospital will be] an absolutely independent entity, an independent company with an independent board . . . it will not be entrusted to the Sisters of Charity in any way.'

Apart from their owning it 100 per cent, that is.

In an opinion piece in the *Irish Times* Nicholas Kearns described some of my statements as 'wild allegations', and also described my call for the building of a hospital on land adjacent to St Vincent's, purchased if necessary by CPO, as showing 'a disconnect from reality that is frankly worrying'.

I hadn't resigned from the board of the NMH, but I slept little that night, and at 5 a.m. I got up and wrote my resignation letter:

I can no longer remain a member of a board which is so blind to the consequences of its decision to transfer sole ownership of the hospital to the Religious Sisters of Charity, and so deaf to the disquiet of the public it serves . . . To believe that the New National Maternity Hospital will be the only hospital in the world owned by a Catholic congregation to permit sterilization, IVF, abortion, gender-reassignment surgery and any other procedures prohibited by the Church is naive and delusional . . . That approximately €300 million of public money will be spent on such a project is a scandal.

I concluded: 'I am saddened to end my association with the hospital to which I have dedicated my professional career in this way.'

I phoned the producer on Newstalk's *Pat Kenny Show* and told her that I would appreciate an opportunity to speak with Pat that morning. She accepted immediately. I did not tell her I had resigned, as I wanted to ensure that Nicholas Kearns heard the news first from me.

On air I said: 'I think it's a scandal that in 2017 the state is going to gift to a religious organization a national maternity hospital, of all things. I really do not think that's acceptable.' I noted that my view was 'shared by an enormous number of people in the country'.

Adrenaline propelled me through the interview with Pat, but, as I talked about how sad I was to end my association with Holles Street in this way, my voice broke with emotion. Pat immediately ended the interview and went into a break. When I got outside the studio, the programme team were solicitous, offering tea, cake and hugs, and giving me time to recover myself.

Resigning from the board of the NMH was the saddest day of my career. I had been involved with Holles Street for nearly forty-four years, since I entered its doors as a medical student in 1973. I had been its master, and later its clinical director for another five years, from 2009 to 2014. I had also served on the board from the time I completed my mastership in 1998.

After I resigned I told Justine McCarthy that I couldn't go to my grave knowing that I didn't do what I should have done. In calling for my resignation there had been an emphasis on my lack of loyalty to the board. This is one of the problems in corporate governance in this country. Board members need to be able to ask difficult questions. If a proposed course of action has serious implications for the people the board serves, then it is a board member's duty to raise this. And if these concerns are ignored, the issue should be brought to public attention. In the case of Holles Street, I believe board members serve the patients and potential patients of the hospital, not each other.

If the boards of the two hospitals thought that after my resignation the matter would settle and they could go back to business as usual, they were to be disappointed. If anything, my resignation added fuel to the fire. I was overwhelmed with messages of support from members of the public, former patients, politicians, colleagues (including from within the NMH) and the media. Drivers in passing cars and buses beeped and waved. People went up to me in the street, and in shops and restaurants, to thank me for what I was doing and to urge me to keep going. There was international media interest. The *Guardian* described my resignation as 'the latest flashpoint in a row that has reignited a debate about church–state relations and the influence of Roman Catholic institutions on the provision of public services'. Taoiseach Enda Kenny was asked to comment on my resignation at a meeting of EU leaders in Brussels. In the *Irish Daily Mail* columnist Philip Nolan captured the general sentiment when he wrote: 'Why is our country so medieval when it comes to silencing dissent? . . . What this suggests to me is that the board is filled with professionals who, outside of the medical environment where their decisions go largely unchallenged, do not seem to realise that a second opinion is welcomed by the rest of us, even if our impertinence chills them to the marrow.'

Inevitably, the family connection excited some in the media. Photographs of Jane appeared in the papers with speculation about relations between her and Rhona, and how our next Christmas dinner might go. Even our dog got a mention. This was unfortunate and uncomfortable, but no more than a sideshow that we could ignore.

The Uplift petition urging the government to reconsider the relocation plan exceeded 104,000 signatories, and there were more protests and demonstrations.

Professor John Crown, who has had well-documented battles with SVHG, said that '[T]he understandable desperation of Holles Street to see this through weakened their negotiating position. I will charitably invoke this weakness as mitigation for their inexcusable abandonment of Dr Peter Boylan following his public articulation of entirely justifiable concerns about the implications of the Sisters of Charity ownership of the NMH.'

Professor Chris Fitzpatrick resigned from the HSE's planning board, noting that '[W]hat is happening has unfortunate resonances of Dr Noël Browne versus Archbishop John Charles McQuaid and the Mother and Child Scheme of the 1950s – and sadly we know how that worked out for Irish women.'

Two former masters of the Rotunda spoke out. Michael Darling said that he was concerned and felt strongly about the issue. 'Regard-less of the reassurances that have been given, it is not a cut-and-dried arrangement. There is a grey area about the governance . . . I believe ownership of the new hospital should be given to the NMH.' Sam Coulter-Smith said I had been absolutely right to speak out. 'There cannot be outside interference with the hospital from any organisation. You can get all the reassurances in the world but once you are in new governance arrangements you don't know how it's going to work.'

In the days following my resignation, the media expanded their investigations, particularly into the question of land ownership and St Vincent's financial arrangements.

Irish Times opinion editor John McManus wrote, 'If the NMH should fear anyone it is not the Sisters of Charity but the lay people they are leaving control of the SVHG to. If they were all Knights of Columbanus or similar hard-core Catholics, then perhaps the fears of Peter Boylan and other opponents of the move might be justified. But a quick look through the board indicates that a common thread run-ning through it is much more likely to be corporate finance rather than Opus Dei.'

While I believed McManus was underestimating the role conserv-ative Catholicism was playing in SVHG's conduct, his drawing of attention to its potentially complicated business arrangements was welcome.

On 29 April, Kieran Mulvey confirmed the complex nature of SVHG's financial and legal arrangements to the *Irish Independent*, one consequence of which was that it would not be possible to cede own-ership of the land at this stage. 'They have other loans . . . The campus as a whole would lose value if a particular section at the centre of it was not under the current arrangement. There are large borrowings of the SVHG which will have to be met.'

I reacted immediately. 'They [the government and parties to the agreement] are saying the state has a lien on the land but how does that work if, as it appears, there is already a lien on the land?'

On Sunday, 30 April, it was reported that the government was exploring the possibility of a 999-year lease on the land to secure state ownership.

On the same day Kieran Mulvey said that the Sisters of Charity would be considering the land ownership issue as part of their operations and went on to criticize the intervention of the former masters of national maternity hospitals in the debate, saying they were speaking about hospitals they no longer had any involvement with or clinical role in. This was unwarranted. I was both a governor of the NMH and a member of the board up to a few days before, and had only retired from clinical practice at the end of 2016. Sam Coulter-Smith's term as master of the Rotunda ended in December 2015, and he was (and is) very much still active in clinical practice, as was (and is) Chris Fitzpatrick at the Coombe.

After the Cabinet met on 2 May, a senior government source told the *Irish Times* that 'it was inevitable the ownership of the hospital would be changed. It is most likely a long-term lease will be entered into in return for a nominal fee to the Sisters of Charity.'

There was now considerable media focus on the ownership of Catholic hospitals. In the *Sunday Times* Justine McCarthy wrote that '[T]he Bon Secours order, which managed the Tuam mother and baby home, has transferred the ownership of its hospitals into a canonical and civil entity, bequeathing them to the bishop of Cork and Ross if the order ceases to exist.' (Six months later, the Sisters of Mercy in Cork incorporated a new organization called Mercy Care South. Its five directors were members of the Sisters of Mercy and its charter stated that '[G]overnance will be conducted in accordance with the teachings of the Catholic Church, the principles of Catholic healthcare and in the spirit of Catherine McAuley, foundress of the Sisters of Mercy.')

The following weekend, Tom Lynch, chairperson of the Mater in Dublin, approvingly described how Belfast's Mater Hospital managed its religious ethos while being funded by the NHS since the early 1970s. 'The government of Northern Ireland undertook, in exchange for a long leasehold of the hospital, to respect and observe its ethos . . . Some forty-five years later the Mater in Belfast adheres to its Catholic ethos and serves the people of Belfast on the basis of need. The vision of Catherine McAuley is as important today as it was 200 years ago.'

To me this appeared as clear advocacy for a Catholic ethos in public hospitals by the man who also chaired the Ireland East Hospital Group. I did not find this reassuring.

In an opinion piece in the *Sunday Business Post* the following weekend I reiterated the known position of Catholic hospitals world-wide and analysed the proposed governance arrangements. I pointed out that 'it would only take one or two future NMH board members to come under the influence of an organization like, for example, Opus Dei, for the whole edifice to come crashing down.'

I noted that Lynch had said that '[W]hen the Mater tendered for the national paediatric hospital to be located on the grounds of the Mater, the order donated the site, free and unencumbered, to the HSE, a gift then valued at €90 million.' The *Sunday Business Post* edited out my next paragraph, in which I asked: 'Could the Sisters of Charity be equally generous? My understanding is that the Sisters own Elm Park Golf Club and Caritas beside St Vincent's. A portion of those lands could be donated or sold to the state and the new NMH could be built and linked to St Vincent's without the need for what Olivia O'Leary recently described on RTÉ radio as the "Byzantine" arrange-ments of the Mulvey Report. A long-term lease would not address the issue of canon law. Discussion of a lien is surely moot given Bank of Ireland already holds a lien on the SVHG campus following the mortgaging of the public hospital to build the private hospital.'

I concluded that '[I]t is therefore clear that ownership, both of the land and the hospital itself, is the crucial issue from which all else flows. The only viable solution would appear to be the construction of the new NMH on land adjacent to, or in very close proximity to, SVH but not owned by the Sisters of Charity.'

On the morning of Monday, 29 May 2017, Gabriel Daly of the Association of Catholic Priests wrote a letter to the *Irish Times*, a shorter version of a blog he had written some weeks earlier. I found Fr Daly's words reassuring. He criticized, with some justification, the 'hostile and sometimes vitriolic' terms used to describe the Sisters of Charity despite their long and valued contribution to the Irish health service. He acknowledged that 'those with more considered reasons feared that there might be interference with medical decisions on reli-gious grounds. This was a fair point usually made by professionals like Dr Peter Boylan, who had the grace to argue temperately and con-vincingly. I find myself convinced by his wise and temperate words.'

Fr Daly had hoped that 'the Church might try to pour oil on troubled waters', but this hope was 'dashed by the entry of the Bishop of Elphin into the affair. His words conjured up the age where the

Catholic Church ruled with confident doctrinal and moral sovereignty and laid down the law in the full expectation of being obeyed without question.' (I would remember these words a year later during the referendum to repeal the Eighth.)

A couple of hours after I read Fr Daly's letter, there came a dramatic development. Sr Mary Christian, congregational leader of the Religious Sisters of Charity, announced that the order would 'end our involvement in St Vincent's Healthcare Group and will not be involved in the ownership or management of the new National Maternity Hospital'.

She said that ownership of SVHG would be transferred to a newly formed company with charitable status to be called St Vincent's. In what appeared to be a highly significant move, Sr Mary announced that 'Upon completion of this proposed transaction, the requirement set out in the SVHG constitution to conduct and maintain the SVHG facilities in accordance with the Religious Sisters of Charity Health Service Philosophy and Ethical Code would be amended and replaced to reflect compliance with national and international best practice guidelines on medical ethics and the laws of the Republic of Ireland.' This was extraordinary. If this promise was to be carried through, canon law would no longer dictate medical practice at SVHG.

I described the move as noble, brave and honest. The religious order, in my view, deserved full credit for the decision to relinquish ownership of the hospital to which they had devoted their lives over more than 180 years, but they should not have been put in such a position in the first place.

The Minister for Health described the announcement as 'truly historic', and it was evident that the government felt, with relief, that enough had been done to defuse the controversy. The *Irish Times* described the order's move as 'a watershed moment in relations between Catholic Church institutions and the State'.

However, I observed with interest the reaction of St Vincent's and Holles Street, somewhat lost as it was in the atmosphere of euphoria and relief. James Menton insisted that '[T]he idea that they were forced into this is a complete misrepresentation of the facts. They didn't ring me two weeks ago and decide this is what they wanted. This takes months of planning.'

I looked for some movement on the governance structure, but there was none. In an *Irish Times* report James Menton simply reiterated that the master of the NMH would report to the group clinical director at St Vincent's following its transfer, rather than to the board of the NMH – exactly as outlined in the Mulvey Report. The fine distinction that a SVHG spokesperson made in the report – that the master would be so reporting only in her role 'as clinical director for obstetrics and gynaecology on the Elm Park campus' of St Vincent's – was moot. The proposed reporting structure fundamentally changed the nature of the master's role and where meaningful power lay.

As for ownership, Menton was clear that the argument that because the state was building the new hospital it should own it, was 'inaccurate' and 'facile', particularly given that St Vincent's was providing a site worth 'tens of millions of euro' and the NMH would be contributing the proceeds of the sale of Holles Street to the building of the new facility. He insisted that for the project to proceed it needed to do so in accordance with the Mulvey Report, and St Vincent's needed to have full ownership of the new NMH in order to ensure there were integrated systems of clinical and corporate governance on its campus.

So, despite everything, Menton was insisting that the Mulvey agreement still held. I concluded that St Vincent's were now showing some desperation in wanting the new NMH. They had walked away from the project several times, but always returned to the table. No matter how bad the publicity, they appeared to grit their teeth and accept it. Now the Sisters of Charity were to walk away from the hospital founded by the remarkable Mother Mary Aikenhead in 1833, the first hospital in Britain and Ireland to be organized and staffed by women.

Since the Catholic ethos issue appeared to have been cleared up, public and media attention shifted to the governance issues. SVHG and Holles Street repeated the same old discredited line about the reserved powers, insisting, in the face of what was written in black and white in the Mulvey Report, that the master would report to the NMH board. I told the *Irish Times* that there was nothing to support this and that 'the Mulvey document is crystal-clear that the master reports to the SVHG clinical director – as confirmed by Mr Menton.'

Though all the discussion seemed to centre on the Mulvey Report, as if it was the final blueprint for the relocation plan, in fact the blueprint was far from fixed. In an *Irish Times* piece in early June I wrote that the Mulvey Report had 'no legal standing in underpinning the proposed move, yet it appears that it is being interpreted by some as binding'. I said that the two hospitals had not even met to discuss drawing up a legal document to advance the move, and the NMH governors had still not been consulted. I pointed out once more that the NMH board – bizarrely and unacceptably – was entirely missing from the clinical governance structure proposed in Mulvey. I concluded by saying '[T]here is clearly massive public support for a truly independent NMH. The decision of the Sisters of Charity opens a window of opportunity to achieve this.'

Yet again Holles Street passed on an opportunity to try to get a better deal for the hospital. The NMH issued a statement that was, forgive the pun, masterly in its confusion of the role of master and clinical director. 'These latest assertions are without foundation. It is being asserted that the master of NMH will report to St Vincent's Hospital in relation to that role. This is false. The master will report to the board of the new NMH in relation to the operation of the hospital, exactly as is the case today. SVHG [has] made clear the master will also fulfil the role of clinical director for obstetrics and gynaecology on the Elm Park campus and will report to SVHG's clinical director in relation to that role only.'

I found this statement bizarre – all anyone had to do was to read through Mulvey to be clear on the real position.

Chris Fitzpatrick told the *Sunday Times* that 'St Vincent's have no record in looking after mothers and babies. I would respectfully suggest SVHG take a leaf out of the Sisters of Charity's book and gracefully withdraw from its insistence on ownership and allow the NMH to retain its voluntary status.'

By now, fortunately, the Minister for Health and the government were fully aware of public opinion. Simon Harris said that '[D]iscussions will, and must, continue to tease out the issues of ownership.' The *fait accompli* so confidently announced by SVHG and the NMH had turned out to be anything but.

On 8 February 2018 Simon Harris told the Dáil that 'there is broad understanding and agreement on the way forward that will protect the State's resources in investing in this important project and it will further underpin the operational independence of the maternity hospital. It is envisaged that the new hospital building will remain in State ownership.' Critically, the new NMH would be listed as an asset on the state's balance sheet, not on that of SVHG. Ellen Coyne reported in the *Times* that '[O]fficials at the Department of Health are said to have planned to use the example of the new maternity hospital as a "roadmap" for separating Church and State in other parts of the health service.'

During 2018 intense negotiations took place between St Vincent's Hospital and the Department of Health regarding alterations to the Mulvey agreement. The key issues were the retention of the ownership of the building of the new NMH by the state and the appointment by the Minister of at least one public interest representative to the board of the new hospital.

A major problem for the Department as the months passed was that there was no movement by SVHG on setting up the new St Vincent's company or applying for charitable status. This was a prerequisite for progress. Worryingly, six months after the sisters' announcement, SVHG included a note in their annual accounts that future directors of the new St Vincent's Company that was to replace SVHG would be obliged to uphold the 'values and vision' of Mother Mary Aikenhead, the founder of the Religious Sisters of Charity. Speaking the following April, the Maynooth theologian Professor Vincent Twomey told the *Sunday Times* that this commitment would require compliance with Catholic medical ethics.

In July 2018 the Irish Catholic Bishops' Conference published its 'Code of Ethical Standards for Healthcare'. The code covered governance and management, directing that '[W]here the ministry of a diocese or religious congregation has been incorporated as a limited company, the board of that company is to act in accordance with its mandate from the diocese or congregation' and that '[C]are must always be taken to ensure that arrangements deriving from contracts with other parties are in accord with Catholic moral and social teaching.'

So Catholic hospitals in Ireland must follow Catholic teaching was the bishops' unsurprising position. The code stated that 'there may be specific procedures which a Catholic healthcare facility cannot provide, by virtue of its ethos', and in a section entitled 'Specific Issues' the code explicitly stated that the following procedures could not be provided by Catholic facilities: any form of artificial contraception, provision of the morning-after pill, any form of assisted fertility treatment, surrogacy, abortion, referral elsewhere for abortion, sterilization and gender-reassignment surgery.

Two months after Ireland had overwhelmingly voted to repeal the Eighth Amendment the Catholic bishops had asserted the Church's right to decide what medical care could be provided in institutions with a Catholic ethos. This made it obvious that for citizens to access all the healthcare options they were entitled to under the law of the land, the Catholic ethos had no place in any hospital built or funded by the state. The bishops' position had the benefit of being clear, unambiguous and true to form. By contrast, whatever was going on with SVHG was anything but clear or unambiguous. Indeed, its position was worryingly opaque.

PART III

15. 'The people will have their say'

For me the campaign to repeal the Eighth Amendment had begun in earnest during the summer of 2017. In April a Joint Oireachtas Committee had been established to consider the Citizens' Assembly recommendations. I was asked if I would appear before it once the parliamentary summer recess was over. Feeling that, at last, there was a genuine window of opportunity for repeal of the amendment, I was more than happy to offer my help. And so, that summer, over the course of long walks in West Cork and along the South Bull Wall in Dublin, I thought about how best to communicate the message that the Eighth was a profoundly hypocritical inclusion in our Constitution and that, above all else, it was harmful and damaging to the women of Ireland.

The Committee, comprising twenty-two TDs and Senators from across the political spectrum and chaired by Fine Gael's Catherine Noone, heard evidence from thirty-four witnesses, as well as representatives from the HSE and relevant government departments. The witnesses were called for their expertise and experience, with Justice Mary Laffoy, who had chaired the Citizens' Assembly, the first one to be called when proceedings began in September. Since the intention of the Committee was purely to gather factual information, no lobby groups were invited to attend, although an exception was made for representatives of the support groups for parents whose children had suffered fatal fetal abnormalities.

I was invited to appear on Wednesday, 18 October, together with Professor Sir Sabaratnam Arulkumaran, the doctor who had chaired the HSE inquiry following Savita Halappanavar's death, and Dr Meabh Ní Bhuinneain from Mayo University Hospital.

The Eighth, I told the Committee that day, was giving rise to significant difficulties for doctors practising in Ireland. It had caused grave harm to women and some had lost their lives because of it. I cited Savita and Miss P as the two outstanding examples of which I had direct experience. Medical personnel, I said, have no difficulties in obeying clear legislation and medical regulations, but we are not trained for the complexities of constitutional interpretation, nor should we reasonably be expected to be when caring for sick women.

I went on to list, starting with the X case in 1992, the various legal cases generated by the Eighth Amendment, explaining to the Committee that behind all the anonymous initials associated with such cases were the difficult and painful real-life stories of Irish women and girls who had to resort to stressful legal processes in the absence of comprehensive legislation on abortion. If the Eighth Amendment was not repealed, I argued, it was inevitable that this list would continue to grow, and Ireland would continue to be subject to censure by international bodies such as the European Court of Human Rights and the United Nations.

I said that the current legal situation was profoundly hypocritical, since our Constitution effectively enshrined a woman's right to commit an act that was a serious criminal offence as long as it was committed outside the state. By any yardstick this was a bizarre situation and a source of embarrassment to many.

By a neat coincidence at the time of the hearing, the female population of the European Union was around 260 million, with 2.6 million, or 1 per cent, of these living in Ireland and Malta. Thus I could tell the members of the Oireachtas that 99 per cent of women and girls in the EU lived in countries where their parliaments had legislated for termination of pregnancy. Other European societies had difficulties with abortion, too – we were far from unique – but their lawmakers had tackled the issue. I thought it anomalous that, while we Irish were enthusiastic Europeans, with polls showing nearly 90 per cent of Irish people committed to membership of the EU, in the matter of women's reproductive health we were outliers in a tiny minority in Europe. Once again, it was my intention to highlight the failure of Irish legislators to do their job.

The key point I had decided to argue to the Committee was that in 2017 the Eighth Amendment was unworkable. Thirty-four years earlier, when it was inserted in the Constitution in 1983, the internet was in its infancy and the abortion pill did not exist. Now, however, we knew that the number of women buying abortion pills online and importing them illegally was on the increase. The genie was therefore out of the bottle in this regard, and doctors were gravely concerned about the potential for harm caused by such unregulated medication. Licensed pills are safe and effective when taken under medical supervision. However, when taken without that oversight, there are significant risks. It was, I felt, a matter of priority, therefore, for the Oireachtas to address the reality of this situation.

The Citizens' Assembly had made a clear recommendation that termination of pregnancy be dealt with by legislation rather than through the Constitution. I told the Committee that I entirely agreed with this, and added that legislation should be supported by regulation by the relevant bodies.

My contribution to the Oireachtas Committee that day distilled all my thinking on the Eighth Amendment to that point. From the beginning of what I knew would be a highly charged campaign, I wanted to provide accurate, detailed and factual information as to how medical practice in Ireland operated under the shadow of the Eighth. It was important to be as clear and open as possible on how the practical implementation of the recommendations of the Citizens' Assembly might be achieved.

It was of huge importance, therefore, that the TDs and Senators understood the question of viability – the stage after which a baby can survive with support outside its mother's womb. In Ireland, a developed country with first-class medical facilities, viability is currently considered to occur at approximately twenty-four weeks gestation. However, some babies born at twenty-three weeks may survive, while others born after twenty-four weeks may not. Among survivors of very premature birth the rate of disability is high, with complications such as cerebral palsy often arising. When obstetricians deliver a baby at the margins of viability, it is standard practice to have a full neonatal paediatric team present to make an immediate assessment about viability and institute intensive care in every case where appropriate.

I told the Committee that I could not envisage a scenario whereby any doctor in Ireland would support any proposal that termination of pregnancy would be contemplated beyond twenty-three weeks. Anti-abortion extremists are known to advance a false narrative on so-called 'late-term abortion', and so I wanted to reassure the Committee on this point.

I turned then to the votes that the Citizens' Assembly had taken in relation to various potential situations, be that where the mother's life was deemed to be at risk, or her health, or where a woman found herself pregnant as a result of rape, or where a fatal fetal abnormality was present.

The vote had been 99 per cent in favour of legalizing termination where the mother's life was at 'real and substantial physical risk'. This had been addressed to a limited extent in the Protection of Life During Pregnancy Act 2013. Despite the warnings by anti-choice campaigners that the floodgates would open, there had been approximately twenty-five terminations each year, and only seven at this point, because of the risk of suicide.

However, a major difficulty with the Act was that it was entirely the responsibility of doctors to determine how close to death, or how sick, a woman had to be before legal termination could be performed. The woman herself had no input into the decision, other than the option of refusing termination and placing her own life at risk. Doctors could be subject to criminal prosecution if it could be established that they had acted in bad faith in recommending a termination, even if the woman herself was happy with the decision. With some 90 per cent of the Citizens having voted in favour of legal termination where there was 'a serious risk' to the health of the mother, I wanted to give the Committee an understanding of how different people quantify or deal with risk.

Serious risk to the physical or mental health of the woman overlaps with threat to the life of the mother because a risk to health may develop into a risk to life. Under the existing legislation doctors had to make judgement calls on the extent of that risk. If they got it wrong, either the mother would die or the doctor would be guilty of committing a criminal offence.

In my submission, therefore, and in later questioning, I explained that there is a great deal of personal interpretation when it comes to assessing risk – what one person may feel is low risk, another may judge to be high. In the context of pregnancy – a very dynamic process where risk can change and the disease process can accelerate very rapidly – I explained that women approach risk in a different way. It was important, I stressed, to take women's viewpoints into consideration, as it is their lives that are the ones at risk.

Some women will risk anything to have a baby. For others, that risk may not be acceptable. But, as the law stood in Ireland in 2017, it was the doctor, not the woman, who had to quantify the risk and determine whether or not it justified a termination of pregnancy.

When it came to the issue of pregnancy as a result of rape, 89 per cent of the Citizens had voted in favour of legal termination, and I suggested to the Committee that such a pregnancy could be dealt with by legislating for the legal prescription of the abortion pill/ medication. Pregnancy tests are now so sensitive that they are positive just before a missed period, and the pills are 99 per cent successful if taken within the first eight weeks.

One point I wanted to make very forcefully in relation to the rape issue was that there is no diagnostic test to confirm rape, and so I strongly recommended that a woman who has undergone that trauma should not be forced to 'prove' rape if she chooses to terminate a resulting pregnancy.

On the question of fetal abnormality that was likely to result in death, either before or soon after birth, the vote showed that 89 per cent favoured legal termination. This issue had been covered at the Committee the previous week by Fergal Malone, master of the Rotunda, and Rhona Mahony, master of the National Maternity Hospital. Both had been very strong on the clinical risks associated with current legislation, primarily because women accessing termination had to travel outside the state. Complications such as haemorrhage could occur during the journey, giving rise to significant clinical risk, and Professor Malone actually referred to a patient from the Rotunda who had died on the journey back from the UK. The threat of criminal sanction, meanwhile, was repeatedly referenced by Dr Mahony.

I entirely concurred with their evidence, pointing out also that women who choose to continue their pregnancies received the full support of a multidisciplinary team, including palliative hospice care for the newborn. The concept of hospice care for the newborn with little or no chance of survival outside the womb was a long-standing practice in Irish neonatal units. It was simply incorrect to state – as anti-abortion campaigners regrettably did – that this care was not available.

My point to the Committee was that in my sadly considerable experience of couples who have the misfortune to receive diagnoses of fetal abnormalities, I have found that some choose to continue with the pregnancy and are much comforted by having some time, however brief, with their baby. In other cases, however, couples feel unable to continue for, perhaps, another several months, and so choose to travel abroad for termination. However, what is not so well understood, I said, is that some couples experience a diagnosis of fetal abnormality on subsequent pregnancies. My experience has been that in the vast majority of these sad cases, the couples choose termination. They simply cannot face the ordeal a second time.

I have also had experience of couples who, prior to screening, declare that they would not seek termination in the event of a serious abnormality being diagnosed, only to change their minds when confronted with the reality of it.

What raised particularly difficult questions was the Citizens' Assembly's vote in relation to a situation where there was significant fetal abnormality that was unlikely to result in death, either before or after birth. The vote here was 80 per cent in favour of termination.

Yet what is a 'significant' abnormality? The 'significance' may depend on the extent of the disability and/or parents' ability to cope with the consequences. In some conditions, particularly genetic, there is a wide spectrum of severity. Again, it is the parents, in consultation with their doctor, who are best able to make decisions in their individual circumstances.

In results that gave rise to the most surprise, 72 per cent of the Citizens voted in favour of legal termination for socio-economic reasons, and 64 per cent voted for access with no restriction. Of those who voted for termination without restriction, 92 per cent voted for a gestational limit of twelve weeks.

It is well documented, I told the Committee, that in countries where abortion is banned, the rate of women dying from unsafe abortion is high, with around 70,000 deaths worldwide each year. It is equally well recorded that countries with liberal laws and easy access to contraception have lower rates of abortion than those with restrictive laws. Women in Ireland with financial resources have access to termination of pregnancy because they can travel to the UK. However, the Ms Y case, among others, had taught me that poor women – those in the care of the state, or refugees, for example – do not have such access. There could be no doubt that without access to abortion in the UK, Ireland would have had an epidemic of illegal abortions and a massive increase in maternal mortality.

The issue of gestational limits was naturally a key issue for committee members. I took the Committee through the positions across the twenty-eight countries of the EU. The limits for termination without (or with limited) restriction vary from ten weeks in the case of Croatia, Portugal and Slovenia to twenty-four weeks in the Netherlands and UK. However, in the majority of countries, the limit is twelve weeks, or ninety days.

I concluded by telling the Committee that I believed that the forthcoming referendum on the Eighth Amendment should put a simple binary question to the electorate – Yes or No to repeal. If repealed, then the detail of legislation would be the responsibility of the Oireachtas.

I thought that the Committee was for the most part notable for its thoughtful and open-minded questioning and collegial atmosphere. It was clear that some members were in favour of repeal and some were opposed, while a third group seemed unsure and undecided.

Although I was clear that to a certain extent doctors have to park their personal views at the door when treating patients, nonetheless two anti-repeal members of the Committee, Senator Rónán Mullen and Deputy Peter Fitzpatrick, tried to concentrate on the personal. Rónán Mullen even went so far as to ask me how many abortions I had performed that were not life-saving for a woman. I declined to answer him, considering it irrelevant and unduly personal when we should have been focusing on women. The answer, incidentally, is zero.

It was also clear that the testimony about Savita had touched a nerve with both Senator Mullen and Deputy Mattie McGrath. In an RTÉ radio interview the next day, however, Senator Mullen crossed a line when responding to Sean O'Rourke's question as to whether Savita would still be alive if she had had a termination when she asked for one. 'If there was abortion on demand she wouldn't have been in hospital because she wouldn't have been pregnant and she wouldn't have been having a miscarriage,' he replied. His clear implication that Savita wanted to abort her pregnancy regardless was so far from the truth and so repugnant that I was surprised O'Rourke didn't pick him up on it.

There was an immediate backlash to Mullen's comments, with Fine Gael TD Kate O'Connell, who was on the show with him, calling them 'disrespectful', while Colm O'Gorman of Amnesty International described them as a 'disgusting slur'. Social media lit up with outrage and disgust.

I wrote to the Oireachtas Committee noting that although Senator Mullen was absent for much of the Committee on other business, while he was present he made several assertions at odds with the facts in respect of my evidence, repeatedly claiming, for example, that Savita's consultant in Galway did not 'hide behind the Eighth Amendment', i.e., that Dr Astbury was in no way constrained by the amendment. I attached, for the Committee's attention, the relevant transcripts from the Galway inquest in which it was abundantly clear from Dr Astbury's evidence that she was indeed constrained by the Eighth.

Since this point was so fundamental to the Committee hearings, I also suggested that the record should be corrected in respect of Senator Mullen's inaccurate assertions. The chair of the Committee agreed that, for the purposes of clarification, my letter and its attachments would be made available on the Oireachtas website and form part of the record of the Committee.

The nature and tone of such erroneous commentary on Savita was an early indication that the circumstances of her death would be misrepresented at every opportunity by those against repeal. It had been apparent to me since the time of Savita's inquest that efforts were being made to portray my opinion as not representative of mainstream medical thinking.

Later in the evening, following our session on 18 October, the Committee took a vote 'not to retain the Eighth Amendment in full'. Fifteen members voted in favour, three against and two abstained. The Committee would now consider six options as alternatives to the Eighth, including its deletion.

That same evening, Taoiseach Leo Varadkar told *Spotlight* on BBC Northern Ireland that he believed there was a strong majority in the country in favour of liberalizing the law, and I felt optimistic that there was real momentum building towards the possibility of a referendum in the next year or so.

★

When the Committee published its 36-page report two months later, outlining the conclusions they had reached and providing background on how they had reached them, it was clear that, although they had considered the recommendations of the Citizens' Assembly, they had come to different views on how repeal might be effected, and on gestational limits.

The key recommendation was that the Eighth Amendment be repealed *simpliciter* – i.e., removed from the Constitution in full. The Citizens' Assembly had rejected simple repeal in favour of replacing Article 40.3.3 with a constitutional provision giving exclusive authority to the Oireachtas to legislate on the issue of abortion, free from the legal uncertainty of constitutional challenge. The Oireachtas Committee, however, disagreed on this point, considering that in the context of the separation of powers in the Irish system of governance it was a step too far to remove the supervisory jurisdiction of the courts.

A second key recommendation was that termination of pregnancy be permitted up to twelve weeks, with no restriction as to reason, while a third advocated for termination in the case of fatal fetal abnormalities. Furthermore, the report made clear that it would be the job of the government to set gestational limits, guided by best medical practice.

In her foreword, Chairperson Catherine Noone summarized the general sentiment of the Committee:

The main conclusion of our work is that we need some change and in order to effect that we need to amend the Constitution to remove article 40.3.3. After many years of public and political debate on the issue, the people will have their say . . . The key change we want to make is to modernise healthcare by placing the woman at the centre of it. What I have learnt over the last three months is that every situation is unique and the evidence has shown that medical practitioners do not feel supported by the law in providing necessary care for the women of Ireland. Women have felt the need to look into different options – travel and more recently the availability of illegal abortion pills [have] come into focus and we cannot continue to ignore this.

The three dissenting members of the Committee, Senator Mullen and the TDs Mattie McGrath and Peter Fitzpatrick, refused to sign the report and issued their own report criticizing the 'unacceptably flawed process' that had led to 'cruel and unjust recommendations'. As the weeks had progressed at the hearings, they had become increasingly disruptive, being rude to witnesses, and staging walkouts and other stunts, usually timed for the early-evening news. They also began to claim that witnesses were one-sided in favour of repealing the Eighth, or 'pushing abortion', as they put it, prompting me to reflect that it was not the witnesses who were taking a particular side, but that the solid evidence was pointing one way. Their behaviour was a concerted attempt to delegitimize the work of the Committee.

After the publication of the report, Taoiseach Leo Varadkar and the Fianna Fáil leader, Micheál Martin, said they would study it over the Christmas break. It would then be discussed at the first Cabinet meeting of the New Year.

I was confident that, after all that had happened in the previous five years – the death of Savita and the reports into her death, the Protection of Life During Pregnancy Act 2013, the cases of Ms Y and Miss P, the recommendations of the Citizens' Assembly in 2017, and now the Report of the Oireachtas Committee on the Eighth Amendment – the government would have no choice but to hold a referendum. I was looking forward to it.

16.   A referendum is announced

At the start of 2018 it was clear that the window of opportunity for repealing the Eighth was finally wide open. As chair of the Institute of Obstetricians and Gynaecologists, I wanted to establish the Institute as an authoritative and expert voice in what was likely to be a difficult, passionate and potentially very divisive national debate. I believed we had a responsibility to provide education and leadership as the relevant specialist body. Not only would this assist with an informed referendum debate, but it would put the Institute in a good position to advocate for the full spectrum of women's healthcare in the future.

Traditionally most Irish obstetricians and gynaecologists are also members of the Royal College in London (RCOG), established in 1929. The IOG was founded in 1968, and there is a widespread view that it was driven by a group of conservative Catholic consultants as a counter to the perceived liberalism of the RCOG in the aftermath of the UK Abortion Act of 1967. The chair in 1983 was Dr Stanley Hewitt of Portiuncula Hospital, one of the PLAC founders. He had trained in the UK, but left the NHS because, as his obituary in 2009 in the *Irish Medical Times* noted: '[H]is Catholic principles prevented him from carrying out some of the procedures that were considered normal for gynaecologists in the UK.'

I knew that there would be differences of opinion among colleagues. Some older retired members had been founder members of the Pro Life Amendment Campaign, and thirty-five years later were as vehemently in favour of the Eighth as they had been in 1983. On the other hand, it was clear that younger doctors and trainees, some of whom had not been born at the time of the previous referendum, overwhelmingly supported repeal. These would be the doctors in practice in the coming decades.

Somewhere in the middle were a number of colleagues who had surprised me during the Citizens' Assembly and Oireachtas Committee deliberations by expressing the view that the debate was of no interest or concern to them. Even more surprising: some of these colleagues were women. Irrespective of their views, they were detached from the debate, seeing it, I think, as a political or legal matter – a 'women's rights issue' – that did not concern them in their day-to-day medical practice. Perhaps it was relevant that the political impetus for repeal had come from the Labour Party, which had opposed the amendment in 1983, and from radical left-wing politicians, not the natural milieu of many Irish medical consultants.

In 1983 the members of the Institute had been deeply divided on the Eighth and unable to reach consensus. There had been near-violent scenes, indeed, at an EGM in July 1983. I wanted to ensure that the acrimony of the previous referendum campaign was avoided, and that the Institute stay united this time, notwithstanding individual differences of opinion.

The business of the Institute is conducted by the executive council, to which all maternity hospitals and units in the country nominate representatives. I convened a special meeting on Monday, 8 January, to discuss the Oireachtas Committee recommendations. Nineteen members out of the twenty-five on the executive were present, providing a good representative turn-out, and the discussion was open and cordial. Colleagues raised concerns about the likelihood of a divisive referendum campaign and discussed the implications for medical practice if the amendment was repealed, and what the legislation to replace it might look like. A vote was taken and eighteen out of the nineteen present voted in favour of supporting repeal. There was one abstention. We came up with a brief statement to reflect the decision: 'The Institute of Obstetricians and Gynaecologists supports the recommendation of the Joint Committee on the Eighth Amendment to the Constitution that Article 40.3.3 be removed from the Constitution. The Institute looks forward to continuing to assist in informing legislation to enhance women's health and safety.'

The statement was circulated to all 200 or so members of the Institute before being issued, generating twenty-three responses. Seventeen endorsed it without reservation, two were non-committal and four opposed it, including three former chairs of the Institute during the 1970s and 1980s – Professor John Bonnar of Trinity College Dublin, Dr James Clinch, former master of the Coombe, and Dr Conor Carr, formerly of Portiuncula Hospital. Their opposition came as no surprise, given their long and sincerely held views.

The IOG meeting had been timed to anticipate the first Cabinet meeting of the New Year, on Wednesday, 10 January. I thought it important that Ministers should know in advance that the professional body representing obstetricians and gynaecologists supported repeal, and so we released the statement publicly on our website, and to the media and all members of the Oireachtas on the morning of the Cabinet meeting.

Our own uncontroversial meeting, with its clear expression of support for repeal, was very different to the position thirty-five years earlier. Dr Michael Solomons of the Rotunda, a founder of Ireland's first family planning clinic, gave a vivid account of the bitter row in the early 1980s in his book *Pro Life? The Irish Question*. He described the history of the Pro Life Amendment Campaign, founded in April 1981 by a group of conservative Catholic doctors to campaign against the possibility of a Supreme Court ruling in Ireland, similar to that of *Roe v. Wade* in America, which had ruled in 1973 that abortion was a fundamental human right. The PLAC's goal was the insertion of an amendment into the Constitution that would copper-fasten a near-total ban on abortion in Ireland.

Michael Solomons was one of the founders of the Anti-Amendment Campaign in May 1982 and had been greatly influenced by his experience at the Rotunda as a young doctor. This was when he first encountered the 'grand multiparas', a term coined in Dublin for women who had seven or more pregnancies. He saw a 26-year-old woman on her sixth pregnancy go blind, only to return pregnant again the following year. In three years in the late 1940s, he recorded, twenty-three women and 800 babies died at the Rotunda. The numbers were similar at Holles Street and the Coombe. Continual child-bearing could have appalling consequences for women's health. 'For them,' wrote Solomons, 'pregnancy was to be a death sentence.' As no mechanical method of preventing conception was available, he recalled, people improvised. A colleague of his attended the birth of a baby with the cap of a Guinness bottle on his head. The mother had hoped it would act as a contraceptive.

A week before the 1983 referendum the *Irish Times* published a story on the death of Sheila Hodgers in Our Lady of Lourdes Hospital in Drogheda. She had been denied treatment for cancer because the hospital's Catholic code of ethics did not permit treatment that could harm the fetus, including either chemotherapy or early delivery, which they considered to be abortion. Mrs Hodgers died in extreme agony from multiple cancers in March 1983, two days after giving premature birth to a daughter who did not survive. Despite her story being made public, the referendum to insert the Eighth Amendment into the Constitution passed by 67 per cent to 33 per cent. Only five constituencies out of forty-one across the country voted against the Eighth: Dublin North-East, Dublin South, Dublin South-East, Dublin South-West and Dun Laoghaire.

If the position of most doctors had changed since 1983, it was clear that there had also been a change in the political weather. It was reported that, following a two-hour discussion in early January 2018, the Cabinet was 'cautiously supportive' of preparing legislation to legalize abortion up to twelve weeks. To the dismay of some supporters of repeal, Taoiseach Leo Varadkar was quoted as saying that the twelve weeks proposal 'might go one step too far' for the public. Less frequently quoted, however, was the fact that he had added: 'But then again, perhaps not. That's the debate we are going to have over the next few months.'

Leo Varadkar was proceeding slowly and carefully. He refused to give his personal views on the Eighth Committee's recommendations at that point, stating that he wanted to study their report and get the views of the Fine Gael Parliamentary Party before commenting. In the *Sunday Independent* that weekend political scientist Eoin O'Malley articulated exactly my own analysis: 'I think Varadkar wants to appear that he is still struggling with the issue. This will make people who are themselves struggling with the question more inclined to listen to him when he comes out and says that he thinks the only way we can deal with the tragic cases the amendment has caused is to repeal the amendment and use legislation.'

A few days after the Cabinet meeting Health Minister Simon Harris invited me to a meeting with the Chief Medical Officer and Department officials. A three-day debate in the Dáil was scheduled to begin the following day, and the Minister wanted a briefing from the Institute. Dr Cliona Murphy of the Coombe, who would succeed me as chair in September, also attended. We had been working in tandem since her election as chair-designate three months earlier to ensure continuity beyond my term. The Minister requested ongoing assistance with the drafting of the legislation, agreeing with us, as he said, that doctors should provide leadership in this referendum campaign. The practice of obstetrics had been tied up in legal and theological arguments since the introduction of the Eighth. It was time now for doctors and women to have their say about the reality on the ground.

In the Dáil debate that commenced on 17 January, Simon Harris focused on that reality, observing that, in 2016, some 3,265 Irish women travelled to the UK (meaning that this number had given Irish addresses). 'These are not faceless women,' he said. 'They are our friends, neighbours, sisters, cousins, mothers, aunts, and wives.' Legislators, he said, would have to take action, given the increase in abortion pills purchased illegally over the internet.

'Research shows a 62 per cent increase in the number of women from Ireland contacting one online provider over a five-year period, from 548 in 2010 to 1,438 in 2015 . . . Can we just pause and picture what this is telling us? Is it acceptable to any of us that women are once again left in a lonely and scary place sending off for a pill to be sent through the post instead of being able to access the medical advice and support they need? This is happening in Ireland today . . . If it is the sad reality that we have been exporting this issue, are we now accepting that women must import their own solutions?'

Overall, a majority of members of the Dáil spoke in favour of repeal during the debate over five sessions. The *Irish Times* noted that 76 TDs were on the record as supporting repeal – 2 short of a simple majority – while 32 were opposed and 50 were undeclared.

On the second day of the debate Micheál Martin made a decisive contribution, declaring that he would vote for the proposal to legalize abortion on request up to twelve weeks. As Martin had previously described himself as a supporter of the constitutional ban on abortion and coming from a 'pro-life' perspective, his announcement stunned many, particularly those in his own party. It was a significant moment and I have no doubt that it had a major impact in moving voters to a position where a vote for repeal was an acceptable option for 'middle Ireland'.

I listened to him on RTÉ's *Morning Ireland* the next day and thought him sincere in describing how his views had evolved. 'The Eighth Amendment,' he said, 'is really inflexible . . . in situations like fatal fetal abnormality.' He said he had been persuaded by the strength of the arguments at the Oireachtas hearings, especially by the reality of the prevalent use of abortion pills; the case of Savita Halappanavar had also had an impact. He added that he trusted obstetricians and women.

It was a deft political move, given that the Taoiseach had not yet stated his position publicly. Nonetheless, Martin deserved enormous credit for taking such a courageous step so early in the debate.

A Cabinet meeting was scheduled for Monday, 29 January, to discuss the timing and wording of the referendum. Cliona Murphy, Fergal Malone and I prepared a Question and Answer press release for circulation that morning to the Oireachtas and the media, addressing the diagnosis of fetal abnormality. Misinformation was beginning to circulate about screening for disability, particularly Down Syndrome. There was a concerted effort by the anti-repeal side to claim that diagnostic tests for genetic anomalies could be reliably performed before twelve weeks, and that this would lead to an increase in abortions for Down Syndrome. Apart from the unpleasant subtext that most, or even all, women would terminate their pregnancies if they found out they were carrying a baby with Down Syndrome, this was a clear attempt to confuse screening with diagnosis.

We laid out the facts clearly. The non-invasive pre-natal test (NIPT) is a screening test that analyses fetal DNA in the mother's blood stream. It can be performed only from nine weeks of pregnancy onwards. As there is no facility in Ireland to analyse the samples, they are sent to the UK or the US. Results are generally available within two weeks. The result does not give a diagnosis, but indicates the chance of chromosomal abnormality. A further test is required to make an actual diagnosis. A specialized analysis for conditions such as Edwards, Patau and Down syndromes takes three to five working days, and the results are then sent back to Ireland. So, a full chromosomal result takes nearly three weeks at a minimum.

We noted that the website for one of the companies that carries out the NIPT cautioned that '[N]o irreversible pregnancy decisions should ever be made' based on the screening result alone. It was therefore clear, we explained, that diagnosis of chromosomal abnormality, while technically possible, can rarely be achieved before twelve weeks. To suggest therefore that disability would be eliminated by enacting legislation in line with the recommendations of the Oireachtas Committee was misleading. The important distinction of screening versus diagnosis was consistently misrepresented by the anti-repeal side in the coming months.

On 29 January the Cabinet agreed to hold a referendum in early summer to 'repeal and replace' the Eighth Amendment. Abortion without indication as to reason would be permitted up to twelve weeks. After that it would be allowed only 'in exceptional circumstances' where there was a 'serious' risk to the life or health of the mother or where there was fatal fetal abnormality. The Minister for Health, Simon Harris TD, would draft a referendum bill for publication in early March.

The Taoiseach commented, quoting President Bill Clinton, that he wanted to see abortion in Ireland made 'safe, legal and rare'. Passing the referendum, he said, meant that Ireland would 'come of age'. We would no longer be exporting our problems. I was especially pleased to note that he said it was 'time to trust women'.

I was optimistic, confident even, that the Eighth Amendment would be repealed. My experience of listening to women over the years had taught me that they were angry about the way they had been treated in Ireland over decades and wanted change. Patients, friends and strangers had consistently encouraged me to keep speaking out against restrictions on women's reproductive rights that left them feeling like second-class citizens. The Citizens' Assembly recommendations had confirmed my view that when people are educated about the realities for women of restrictive laws on reproduction, they understand the need for a nuanced and compassionate approach. The result of the 2015 referendum on marriage equality had encouraged me in my optimism that Ireland was a very different country to that of 1983.

Despite Cabinet agreement, a potentially serious political problem arose the following day, when, on RTÉ radio, Tánaiste Simon Coveney said that, while he supported repeal, he could not support the proposal for unrestricted abortion up to twelve weeks. He spoke repeatedly of the need to 'protect an unborn child' and proposed a system whereby a woman who was raped could be 'quickly referred to an individual doctor' from a panel of registered GPs who had 'expertise in the area'.

Such a proposal was unworkable, and David Kenny, assistant professor of Law at Trinity College, who had given evidence to the Eighth Committee, stated in a newspaper interview that, legally, it raised significant problems. 'Essentially, it asks doctors to decide upon a factual and legal question – has rape occurred? – rather than a medical matter.'

Dr Maeve Eogan of the Rotunda's sexual assault treatment unit (SATU) asked what would happen if the GP said no?

Coveney's suggestion would have put doctors back into the position we were trying to escape from: making legal rather than clinical judgements when dealing with patients.

While the Tánaiste's position seemed to be a major set-back, it had the benefit of focusing the spotlight on just why the Eighth Committee had reached consensus on termination without reason up to twelve weeks – there was no feasible alternative to deal with rape, incest and the increasing importation of illegal pills. His public agonizing probably reflected the uncertainty of many. When it became clear that he could not suggest a workable solution, I think many people came to the same view. Some weeks later Coveney announced he would support the twelve weeks legislation.

On Thursday, 8 March – International Women's Day – Minister Harris confirmed that the Cabinet had approved the Thirty-sixth Amendment of the Constitution Bill 2018 and published the draft legislation. Having advised the Minister and the Department over the previous two months, alongside Cliona Murphy, I had reviewed it the day before. A major concern for the Institute was the increasing importation of abortion pills and their use without medical supervision. We were aware of a woman who had recently suffered a uterine rupture in these circumstances, and instances of this potentially serious complication were only likely to increase. Having discussed it with some colleagues, I had written to the Minister stating that the Institute recommended the licensing and regulation of these medications in the interests of women's safety. This would only be possible, of course, if the Eighth were repealed.

Another major concern was the question of fetal viability. In the course of dealings with the Minister I had made it clear that in the case of termination in the interests of a mother's life or health from the point of fetal viability onwards, then the legislation should clarify that it is an 'early delivery'. Thus, as is standard practice now, the full range of neo-natal intensive care services should be deployed if appropriate. Not a single obstetrician in Ireland, I believed, would countenance any other course of action. The Minister and the officials in the Department of Health were in full agreement. The published legislation did indeed contain a clear definition of fetal viability.

Shortly afterwards, I got a phone call from Amy Rose Harte, who introduced herself as the communications director of a campaign for repeal that would be launched by an umbrella group of seventy civil society organizations the following week. She asked if I would attend and give a medical perspective on the Eighth Amendment. I was happy to agree.

When I walked into the Pillar Room at the Rotunda on that Thursday morning, 22 March, however, I had no idea what to expect. The room was crowded with young and energetic volunteers, and there was an electric atmosphere. Simon Harris was there, as were politicians from every party except Fianna Fáil.

The campaign was to be called Together for Yes and included the National Women's Council, the Rape Crisis Network, the Irish Family Planning Association, Women's Aid, the Well Woman Centre, the Union of Students in Ireland, and dozens more. These groups had different perspectives at times, but it was clear they understood the need for a united and broadly based campaign. The campaign's three co-directors were Ailbhe Smyth, a long-time advocate and a convenor of the Coalition to Repeal the Eighth, Grainne Griffin of the Abortion Rights Campaign and Orla O'Connor of the National Women's Council. They made clear that the campaign would be respectful and fact-based, with a focus on 'Care, Compassion and Change'.

I thought the message and the logo were brilliant. There was a clear unity of purpose, and, although I have little knowledge on the subject, I thought the 'branding' was attractive and memorable. Emma Allen of the Abortion Rights Campaign explained that the idea behind the speech bubbles was that conversations were going to be key in the campaign. The aim was to open up conversations in families, in workplaces, in the pub.

Gerry and Gaye Edwards of the Termination for Medical Reasons group (TFMR) spoke movingly about their son Joshua, who had anencephaly, a condition where the brain fails to develop. It is invariably fatal within a short time after birth, usually within minutes. In 2001 they had travelled to Belfast for a termination at twenty-two weeks. Joshua's remains were cremated, and his ashes returned to his parents by courier. Gaye noted that 'couples still have to go through the same trauma, isolation and exile as I did, seventeen years later, it's just not right.' Gaye and Gerry set the tone of the campaign from the beginning: personal stories were key.

When it came to my turn, I spoke about the grave harm the Eighth had caused to so many women and about the risks involved in buying abortion pills online that were being taken without medical supervision. I repeated what I had said at the Oireachtas Committee: the genie is out of the bottle on the pills. We couldn't go backwards. Therefore on voting day it would not be a vote for or against abortion in Ireland – because abortion was already here.

I told the audience that in 1983 the Institute of Obstetricians and Gynaecologists did not have an official position on the Eighth Amendment but that thirty-five years later, having seen at first hand its unintended and unforeseen consequences, the Institute had an agreed position and wanted to see the Eighth repealed.

'Ireland was another country in 1983,' I said. 'I have colleagues who voted for the Eighth in good faith. Having seen the consequences, many tell me they never anticipated how it would work in practice.' This was an important point to make. Two thirds of voters had been in favour of the Eighth in 1983. Many of them would be going to the polls again at the end of May. I wanted them to understand that, even though they had voted for what they considered the best of reasons, the Eighth was harming women.

I addressed the question of fatal fetal abnormalities. Doctors wanted to be able to offer the same pathway of care to parents who chose to go to term with such a pregnancy and to those who felt that, in those circumstances, early delivery or termination was their best option. Under the Eighth we could only help one group. I warned that we could not rely on England as an escape valve forever – we knew that Liverpool Women's Hospital had closed its doors for two weeks earlier in the year to women coming from Ireland, and was now limiting admissions. It seemed likely that as pressure continued on the NHS matters would only get worse. As a mature and independent nation it was time, I said, for us to take responsibility ourselves and repeal the Eighth Amendment.

The retired Supreme Court judge Catherine McGuinness, invited along to give her legal perspective, noted that she had campaigned against the insertion of the Eighth into the Constitution, and that the 'tragic medical cases' of the last thirty-five years had only strengthened her original beliefs. Judges had felt their hands tied by the Eighth Amendment. She said she remembered the misery of the 1983 campaign and hoped this time around it would be respectful and rational.

Most reports of the Together for Yes launch led with my comments about the harm the Eighth was causing women, including death. This was an early signal that the contribution of doctors and medical evidence was going to be significant. I wondered how many doctors would speak publicly. For years it had seemed that Dr Mary Henry, Professor Veronica O'Keane, Dr Mary Favier and I had been alone in speaking on the record about the Eighth. More recently, Cliona Murphy, Rhona Mahony and Fergal Malone had added their voices. A few days after the Together for Yes launch, a doctor at one of the Dublin maternity hospitals lamented to me that 'It seems so few of our profession are willing to be involved, even educationally.'

It is not easy to put your head above the parapet on any issue, let alone one as difficult and controversial as abortion. It was a big step for many colleagues from agreeing that the Eighth should be repealed to talking publicly about their views and experiences. It also seemed that some doctors confused advocating for repeal with advocating for abortion. That wasn't the case: our job as doctors is to give all the facts and information, but we must always let the patient decide what is right for them.

A couple of days after the launch I received a letter from Michael O'Connell, incoming master of the Coombe in January 2020, and Michael O'Hare, who had abstained on the Institute's executive vote in January. They had no issue, they said, with any individual campaigning on either side 'in a private capacity', but '[Should I] choose to continue campaigning for repeal, the way forward from [their] perspective was very clear.' I should stand down as chair of the Institute.

They took issue in particular with my reference to Miss P at the Together for Yes launch. I had indeed discussed the tragic circumstances of Miss P at the campaign launch, and, although the two doctors were 'unsure' if what I had said was in the public domain, they considered 'that use of intimate details of this tragic case in support of the repeal argument in a public forum an abuse of your privileged position as a medical witness. We believe it is unbecoming of the Chairman of the Institute, and unacceptable.' These were strong accusations to make, notwithstanding our differences of opinion on the Eighth.

I replied that as chair of the Institute, I regarded it as part of my duty to provide factual information to any group that requested it. 'Indeed,' I wrote, 'it would be bizarre if the Chair of the Institute of Obstetricians and Gynaecologists were to remain silent on the position of the Institute in relation to repeal of the Eighth Amendment!' Was I to say 'No comment' to questions and requests for information? We were still two months away from the referendum, and it was clear that members of the Oireachtas and the general public wanted to hear from doctors.

Their comments about Miss P were gratuitous, given the widespread media coverage the case had received. Perhaps they didn't understand that open evidence given in the High Court is in the public domain. I had also raised the case at the Eighth Committee in the Oireachtas five months earlier.

As it happened, at a regional meeting a couple of weeks later, where I talked again about Miss P, friends of her family came up to speak to me afterwards. The family knew that I was speaking that day and had asked them to thank me for highlighting her case. They would not be speaking publicly, but they absolutely supported repeal and wanted me to continue.

17. Criss-crossing Ireland to argue for Repeal

On 28 March Simon Harris announced that the referendum would take place on 25 May. The following day the first of the two separate campaigns against repeal was launched. The campaign manager of Save The 8th was Niamh Uí Bhriain, a co-founder of Youth Defence and a member of the anti-abortion lobby group the Life Institute. Its communications director was John McGuirk, formerly of Libertas, a small political party founded by the conservative telecoms entrepreneur Declan Ganley in 2009. Nearly five years earlier McGuirk, as I have described earlier, had disseminated the letter written by a group of anti-choice doctors suggesting that my evidence to Savita Halappanavar's inquest was personal, not professional.

Niamh Uí Bhriain focused her attack on politicians. Politicians were 'effectively seeking a licence to kill', she said. 'The public cannot trust politicians with the right to life in the womb.' Amusingly, in reference to the Tánaiste's changing position, she said that '[T]here have been more flip-flops in the Dáil than on the average beach.'

The anti-repeal obstetrician John Monaghan said keeping Miss P on life support was not at all macabre. 'I thought it was a noble thing although almost an impossibility that the baby could be kept alive until such time it could be able to survive.' He said in the course of delivering up to 5,000 babies during his career the Eighth Amendment had never prevented him from protecting a woman's life. This would become a recurring theme of the doctors who opposed repeal: they had never had a problem with the Eighth personally, ergo there was no problem with it.

The RTÉ *Six One News* phoned me for a comment to fulfil the broadcasting balance requirement. I told them that those who say you should not trust politicians are being 'very anti-democratic', and the approach was 'typical of the alt-right in the US'. I had already noticed on social media that much of the positive response to posts from No campaigners was coming from American accounts. This was to become more noticeable as the campaign progressed.

When I had turned up for the launch of Together for Yes on 22 March, I had not seen myself as 'campaigning' in a political sense. I had based my words that day on my medical experience and would have been more than happy to address groups who opposed repeal, but none invited me to speak. Otherwise the only public meeting I had addressed was a local one in Rathmines at the invitation of Annette Mooney of People Before Profit. I had already spoken publicly, of course, about Savita and Miss P, and I was aware that what I had said had struck a chord publicly. So, while I didn't consider myself a campaigner, when Amy Rose Harte asked me if I would become more involved with Together for Yes, I agreed. Since I had already been accused of 'campaigning', I figured I might as well be hanged for a sheep as a lamb.

As well as Amy Rose, I got to know Deirdre Duffy, the campaign director, and Yvonne Judge, communications strategist, a hugely experienced former journalist and radio producer. Deirdre had been working on the issue for many years, since her time in the Irish Council for Civil Liberties. Yvonne was a veteran of the successful marriage equality campaign three years earlier. It was obvious that the Together for Yes leadership was working to a clearly defined strategy that moved through well-planned phases, with the focus on personal stories and medical advice. Essentially, this was a campaign being run quite brilliantly by an exceptional group of women.

Early and rather trivial media coverage in the second week of April that concentrated on which side had got their posters up first was supplanted by coverage of a successful Together for Yes crowd-funding operation, launched at 8.30 a.m. on Tuesday, 10 April. The initial target was to raise €50,000 in seven days to cover the cost of 5,000 posters. Within two hours that target was exceeded. By 9 p.m. the same evening €250,000 had been raised. Three days later more than €500,000 had been pledged, evidence of both momentum and wide public support.

The campaign strategists wanted me to speak at as many regional meetings as possible, partly to secure regional media coverage, but also so I wouldn't be perceived as someone speaking from an ivory tower in Dublin. I was happy to assist in any way I could. So, with Jane as adviser, sounding board and constant companion, we went to Donegal (three times), Leitrim (twice), Waterford, Athlone, Longford, Galway, Dublin (several meetings) and Sligo. In Dublin, we went to a meeting organized by Joan Burton TD in Castleknock and a ROSA rally in Liberty Hall, where the actress and comedian Tara Flynn and the film director Lenny Abrahamson spoke brilliantly. (Tara was one of a number of high-profile women, which also included the *Irish Times* journalists Róisín Ingle and Kitty Holland, who told their stories of having had abortions. Though these women were somewhat used to being in the public eye, revealing such private and painful experiences was remarkably generous; indeed, their high profiles left them exposed to receiving negative reactions, so their openness was particularly brave.)

The format of the Together for Yes meetings was similar around the country. The aim of the meetings was to foreground the stories of women and couples, and the experience of doctors. Ailbhe Smyth, Grainne Griffin, Orla O'Connor or Sarah Monaghan (a co-convenor of the Abortion Rights Campaign and key member of the Together for Yes team) spoke first on behalf of the campaign. They must have covered thousands of kilometres each but their energy and good humour were undiminished.

I usually spoke next, making the same case over and over again: the vote on 25 May is not a vote for or against abortion, because abortion is already here in Ireland. In 1983 the Institute of Obstetricians and Gynaecologists did not have a position on the Eighth Amendment. Thirty-five years later, having seen at first hand the unintended, unforeseen and harmful consequences, we support repeal. We respectfully ask the Irish people to please vote Yes.

I talked about the risks of importing illegal and unregulated pills. I described how the Eighth had harmed Savita and Miss P, and pointed out that we could change nothing unless the Eighth was repealed. I recalled how it took the death of Savita Halappanavar to bring in the bare minimum of the Protection of Life During Pregnancy Act in 2013, which allowed termination of pregnancy only if a woman might die. I adopted a line from a letter written to the papers by Dr Brendan McDonnell of the Coombe: 'Not dying in pregnancy is the lowest bar we should be aiming for in modern medicine.'

As Jane and I criss-crossed the country, we regularly met Dr Siobhan Donohue, Arlette Lyons, Claire Cullen Delsol, Jennifer O'Kelly, Tracey Smith, and Gaye and Gerry Edwards, all associated with

Termination for Medical Reasons. They retold the stories of coping with devastating diagnoses and then heart-breaking journeys abroad for terminations to highlight the cruelty of what the Eighth had inflicted on them. They were an extraordinary and inspirational group who, since 2012, had fought a lonely battle for recognition of their cause, but now they were central to the debate. The campaign took a heavy toll, but their fortitude and solidarity carried them. Listening to their stories at meeting after meeting was always emotional.

There were light moments alongside the emotional intensity of the meetings. I waltzed down a Galway street with the irrepressible Arlette Lyons. Her parents, Pat and Mary, supported her at meetings, and her father movingly and amusingly expressed his pride in his daughter. The weather in April and May 2018 was beautiful, and driving around the country was a joy. Everywhere we met enthusiastic young volunteers. Their determination to make things right for women and change Ireland was palpable. All told of conversations they were having with parents and grandparents, and on doorsteps around the country. Some of those conversations were difficult, but they persisted. Sometimes, they said, they were pushing an open door.

Most of our audiences were already Yes voters, but there were a number of undecided and No voters at the meetings, too. Generally, they listened with respect to the TFMR parents and asked genuine questions if they spoke at all. A notable exception was a radio debate in Donegal on 11 May organized by Ocean FM, where a group of No voters shouted, hectored and jeered throughout. I joined local activists Trish Hegarty and Cathie Shiels on the Yes side. Lawyer Caroline Simons, Dr Brendan Crowley, a sports GP in Cork, and local activist Mary Stewart spoke for the No side.

Caroline, who, with fellow lawyer Cora Sherlock, had launched a second anti-appeal campaign, Love Both, a month earlier, had driven from Cork through the night to get to the hotel where the debate was taking place. I felt she was feeling the strain of the campaign. Caroline was a fellow governor of Holles Street. We had known each other for many years, and, while we disagreed on the issue of choice, we had a cordial relationship.

Before the debate started, I had a pleasant chat with a Donegal GP who had been in UCD around the same time as me. But all affability disappeared when the debate commenced. Jane had mistakenly sat among the No side of the audience. Following a pretty awful remark by my old colleague, who was sitting behind her, she turned and asked him to stop shouting. He kept going. Three seats from her a middle-aged woman was repeatedly shouting 'murderer' at me. There was little attempt by the producers to rein them in.

After the debate, Caroline Simons went up to Jane. They hugged and both were in tears. Caroline was visibly shocked that day. At one point she had intervened to support my response after a member of the audience claimed, to cheers, that doctors would 'murder' babies up to full term.

Despite that, our campaign memories of Donegal are happy ones. We visited three times and got to know a great group of people who told us that their canvass returns were showing majority Yes voting intentions in many parts of the county.* Similarly, we went twice to Leitrim, where Together for Yes campaigners told us that they were seeing two-to-one Yes returns on their canvasses.† Many older women were saying quietly to them that they were Yes voters but didn't want to speak publicly. This mirrored my own experience. Women had been telling me for years, in the quiet of my consulting rooms, that they agreed with my stance against the Eighth.

As the campaign went on, other doctors came forward, especially Mary Higgins, Rhona Mahony and Venita Broderick of Holles Street, Cliona Murphy, Aoife Mullally and Brendan McDonnell of the Coombe, Louise Kenny, Keelin O'Donoghue, Noirin Russell and Richard Greene in Cork, and Maeve Eogan, Jen Donnelly, Sharon Cooley and Fergal Malone of the Rotunda. Not only did they speak at meetings and to the media, but many of them canvassed

---

* When the results came out, repeal was narrowly defeated in Donegal, the only constituency in the country to vote against repealing the Eighth Amendment. The vote was No 51.87 per cent and Yes 48.13 per cent. However, nine electoral divisions in the south of the county are in the Sligo–Leitrim constituency, where there was a majority vote for Yes.

† The Sligo–Leitrim vote for repealing the Eighth was Yes 59.38 per cent and No 40.62 per cent.

together after long days in the hospital. The GPs Mark Murphy, Anna McHugh and Mary Favier were also tireless.

One of Louise Kenny's patients was Michelle Harte, who had died of cancer in 2010. When she became pregnant, Ms Harte had been in remission for some time after joining a randomized control trial for a new cancer treatment. In a newspaper interview Louise made clear the impact of the Eighth on Ms Harte: 'Michelle's choices were to have a termination of pregnancy and stay on the drug, or not have a termination of pregnancy, but that meant she would have to exit the drug trial at a late stage of malignant melanoma – which was a certain death sentence.' Louise believed that continuing with the pregnancy posed a substantial threat to Ms Harte's life and thus qualified her for a termination here in Ireland, but after two weeks of deliberation Cork University Maternity Hospital's ethics committee disagreed.

Having been ill for some time, Ms Harte did not have a passport, so that delayed things further. Because she had cancer, Ms Harte had to go to a hospital rather than a clinic in the UK to have a termination. But because of the Eighth Louise couldn't communicate with doctors in that hospital about Ms Harte's case.* So, she found herself dealing with a woman with complex medical conditions, and had to tell her that not only could she not treat her in Ireland and she would have to travel abroad, but that she couldn't even pick up the phone on her behalf to refer her – Ms Harte would just have to take her chances.

'Between waiting for the ethics committee to give a decision on whether we could do this in Ireland, and the three to four weeks to get a passport and go to the UK, she was off that trial drug for the whole time and the cancer returned, and she died,' Louise Kenny recalled. 'It goes against everything I've been trained to do as a doctor.'

---

* In the aftermath of the X case in 1992, constitutional amendments allowed doctors to inform women about all their options should they require a termination, and to give them a copy of their notes, but the law prevented us from actually referring them to colleagues in the UK. The women had to make their own arrangements with the clinics and hospitals. This absence of continuity of care was totally contrary to clinical best practice and a source of great anxiety to both patients and doctors.

The No side found fewer doctors prepared to speak. The three most prominent anti-repeal obstetricians were John Monaghan, Eamon McGuinness (both retired), and Trevor Hayes, who was still practising in Kilkenny. On one occasion Eamon McGuinness chaired a meeting for the Save The Eighth campaign where he introduced a woman who said that during her fifth pregnancy she developed life-threatening sepsis, the same condition, Dr McGuinness said, that led to the death of Savita Halappanavar. The patient said that she knew 'from first-hand experience that doctors were not constrained by the Eighth Amendment from acting to save my life'. What the doctor and his patient failed to say, of course, was that the sepsis was in the woman's spine, not her womb, so the Eighth had no relevance.

Meanwhile the Love Both campaign claimed that the proposed legislation was 'more extreme' than that in the UK, which was clearly incorrect, and Cora Sherlock said it was 'a simple option that's on the table for people on 25 May. It's either protect mothers and babies on the one hand, or introduce abortion on demand on the other hand.'

The problem for the anti-repeal campaigns, however, was that as time went on and people understood the issues and heard personal stories, they realized that, far from being 'simple', the situations that women might find themselves in were complex and nuanced. And in such circumstances the No side campaigners had no solutions to offer.

Given the increasing importance of doctors in the campaign, an Institute EGM on 13 April attracted media attention. This had been requested three weeks earlier by a group of consultants at the Coombe, who had proposed the following motion: 'In terms of the forthcoming Referendum, the proposals of the Joint Oireachtas Committee on the Eighth Amendment, the Policy Paper on the Regulation of Termination of Pregnancy approved and published by Government on 8th March 2018, and the proposed legislative changes, that the Institute prepare a position paper based on medical facts and service implications and that any or all communications on behalf of the Institute are based solely on this paper which will be prepared by the membership.'

Since the campaign was well under way at that point, and the Institute's position in support of repeal had been decided in early January, the motion was clearly intended to restrict my ability to advocate for repeal in my role as Institute chair, as I would now have to refer all questions to a position paper. I wasn't going to agree to this, and neither was I going to step aside as chair. As it happened, stepping aside as chair was not part of the motion submitted by the Coombe doctors, and, although it was raised at the meeting, no vote could be taken on it. A constructive discussion took place in a reasonably cordial atmosphere. At the end of the meeting it was agreed to develop position papers on different aspects of the proposed service, and that these would form the basis of future clinical guidelines in the event of repeal.

It seemed to me that the Coombe doctors were narrowly focused on the referendum as an issue for the obstetric profession in Ireland, and perhaps were not considering its broader significance both in Ireland and indeed further afield, where the repeal campaign was seen as a major battle in the global war on women's reproductive rights. Ireland was viewed as the last outpost of Catholic ethos in Europe, and requests for comments and interviews were coming from all around the world. I spoke to the *Wall Street Journal*, several programmes on the BBC, Sky News, the *Guardian*, the Canadian Broadcasting Corporation and the *Lancet*, among others. Or perhaps they could see the resonance this question had outside of our immediate professional concerns, but did not think we should be part of the wider cultural conversation; the professions tend to be cautious about being seen to enter into the grubby political fray (far better to operate in the background). But to me it seemed ludicrous to suggest that the chair of the Institute of Obstetricians and Gynaecologists would not be allowed to advocate for women's reproductive rights. Besides, my colleagues were very familiar with my views when they elected me to the position in 2015.

As referendum day approached, the number of doctors advocating for repeal was growing. A meeting at the Alexandra Hotel in Dublin was attended by several hundred doctors of all ages but with the majority being relatively young. It was clear that there was massive support for repeal from those who were going to be caring for women in the future. The mood of the meeting at a tense time in the campaign was enthusiastic and collegiate, and I found the experience consoling and reassuring.

★

The first televised debate was scheduled for *The Late Late Show* on 27 April, and I was asked to appear with Mary Favier. In putting Mary and me forward, the Together for Yes team was sticking to the strategy of foregrounding doctors in the debate. Around 500,000 people watch *The Late Late* every week, and Together for Yes viewed it as a critical opportunity to get the message out to 'middle Ireland'.

The No side put up the GP Brendan Crowley and Wendy Grace, a presenter on a religious radio station, but Dr Crowley was ill at the last moment and Caroline Simons took his place.

I had three minutes at the beginning of the debate to put the Yes side and I reiterated my points, yet again, that the vote on 25 May was not a vote for or against abortion as it was already here. Over 2,000 women in the previous year alone had imported pills. This, I felt, was a key point to get across; we effectively now had backstreet abortion in Ireland.

I also observed that in 1983 the coalition government's own Attorney General, Peter Sutherland, had argued strongly that the proposed amendment was deeply flawed. He said the wording was 'ambiguous and unsatisfactory' and would inevitably lead to 'confusion and uncertainty', both among doctors and also among lawyers. I knew a lot of older viewers respected Peter Sutherland for his many achievements and also knew that his Catholic faith was important to him. I was making the point that one could be a Catholic but also see the harm of the Eighth.

Two women in the audience told their stories. TFMR's Tracey Smith described how her daughter Grace was diagnosed in the womb with a condition that meant her bones wouldn't grow. This would cause her lungs to be crushed before she reached full term and she would die painfully at birth. Tracey chose to have her daughter delivered at twenty-eight weeks and went to Liverpool Women's Hospital. After a 36-hour labour the baby was delivered still-born. Tracey described how she spent twelve hours with Grace before returning home. She and her husband could not afford to go back to Liverpool for Grace's funeral, and instead were given a tracking number by a courier firm who delivered their daughter's ashes to their home. Tracey appealed to the audience: 'A Yes vote would mean Grace could rest in peace and I would have to stop constantly trying to tell her story.'

On the other side, Mary Kenny described how she had become pregnant at the age of nineteen in her second year in college. Mary was not ready for motherhood and planned to have a termination in England, but a remarkable series of unfortunate events meant that her passport had expired and the abortion pills she ordered online never arrived. Mary was happy to have had her child after all, telling the audience that 'We cannot deny the humanity of the unborn child.'

Together for Yes thought that *The Late Late* was a significant moment in the campaign. Feedback found that Mary Favier and I had been viewed as 'voices of sense'. I was told that I was connecting with voters and having a positive impact. To my amusement, given the feelings of some of my colleagues, I was seen as independent and reassuring to undecided voters. The corollary, I was warned, was that I should expect attempts to undermine me.

In the last ten days of the campaign, three more television debates were viewed as key events. RTÉ's *Claire Byrne Live* was scheduled for 14 May; *Prime Time* for 22 May; and *The Pat Kenny Show* on TV3 was to host the final debate, on 23 May, before the broadcast moratorium kicked in.

Since two men appearing together was obviously not a good idea, the campaign team mulled over whether it would be better for Simon Harris or me to go on *Prime Time*. My contribution to debates was medical and fact-based, and there were worries that *Claire Byrne Live* was a little lightweight for this approach, and, given the live audience and roving-mic format, the debate might turn into a free-for-all. In the end, however, it was agreed that it would be a risk worth taking for me to go on *Claire Byrne Live* with Orla O'Connor of the National Women's Council of Ireland and Sinn Féin's deputy leader Mary Lou McDonald. Simon Harris would go on *Prime Time* with Mary Higgins of Holles Street.

Since joining the campaign Mary Higgins, an expert in complex pregnancies, had been a highly effective speaker. Unlike the doctors on the No side, who claimed never to have had a problem with the Eighth, Mary saw highly complex cases regularly in Holles Street, many of them referred from regional hospitals such as Portiuncula and Kilkenny. This explained, perhaps, how the No side doctors could claim to have no issues with the Eighth.

On the morning of the *Claire Byrne Live* debate a letter from Professor John Higgins and sixteen consultants in Cork University Maternity Hospital and the South/South West Hospital Group asking me to stand down as chair of the Institute was leaked to RTÉ. The first I heard of it was when the RTÉ newsroom rang me for a reaction. The doctors wrote that the consultant body had 'a strong consensus view that the Institute should, as a professional body, reflect the diversity of views [of members] by not campaigning actively for either side'. They recognized that 'individual colleagues' could campaign, but, as I was chair and the 'public face', I should 'refrain from public advocacy'.

It was an illogical position. Every other member of the Institute, including the incoming chair, not to mention former chairs, could campaign on the Institute's agreed position (or against if they chose), but not the current chair.

I wasn't entirely surprised to see some of the names on the letter, but one of the signatories had spoken at the Fine Gael campaign launch in Cork at the end of April. I had written to him after that event to say well done, and how important it was for the public to hear from a variety of doctors. I said that the examples he gave at the launch 'were perfect to illustrate the difficulties with the Eighth'. It was dispiriting, therefore, to see that he had signed the letter.

As it turned out, only nine of the signatories were members of the Institute. Furthermore, Louise Kenny, Keelin O'Donoghue and Noirin Russell immediately contacted me to say that it was untrue to say that there was consensus in the consultant body in Cork. They had known nothing about the letter and disagreed with it. Much like the letter leaked to the Pro Life Campaign after the Savita inquest, none of the signatories could explain how the media got hold of the letter before I had seen it. It was all rather unsavoury, and a bit of a distraction ahead of the debate that night, which was, presumably, the intention.

There was a strategy meeting at Together for Yes HQ before the show. Mary Lou McDonald joined by phone. I had not met her before and was impressed by how well briefed she was and also with her focus on the campaign aims rather than her party political position. When I met her later in RTÉ, I thought she was warm and amusing and rather a good person to have on one's side in a debate. I had got to know Orla over the course of the campaign and knew she would be calm and effective.

I had appeared on television many times. I was familiar with *Prime Time* and had even survived Vincent Browne's tough scrutiny on TV3. So I had a sense of what live television was like. But there was an odd dynamic at play in RTÉ that Monday evening. When Claire Byrne came in to talk to us, she was pleasant and professional but she seemed on edge, even nervous. We were somewhat surprised by the arrival of Dee Forbes, RTÉ's director general, and Jon Williams, its managing director of news and current affairs. Dee Forbes welcomed us quietly, while Jon Williams was talkative and seemed excited. As if in anticipation of difficulties, he said that we would have an open mic to Claire, and that we should signal to her if we needed to respond to a particular point and she would immediately come back to us. Claire herself confirmed this.

Because the No side had two separate campaigns, it was never quite clear in advance who would appear at debates, especially as relationships between the two groups began to deteriorate in the last couple of weeks before the referendum vote. In the end, John Monaghan from Save The Eighth was put forward, together with lawyer Maria Steen of the Iona Institute, and with Fianna Fáil TD Mary Butler as the political representative.

The debate began calmly enough, but soon descended into chaos. There were constant interruptions, and jeering and clapping from the audience. The promise that we could get back in on obviously incorrect statements went by the wayside. When TD Mattie McGrath called me a liar, I asked Claire to be allowed to respond, but she did not give me the opportunity to do so. The No voters heckled and jeered every time I spoke. Several of the hecklers had been at the Ocean FM debate in Donegal three days earlier.

Maria Steen brandished a copy of the legislation and claimed that there was no protection for babies who had reached viability. This was untrue.

I was in a difficult position countering statements from audience members that were clearly medically impossible. As a doctor, I know that people who have had traumatic experiences may have unreliable memories of what happened, but I also know that they believe their memory to be genuine. That was not a discussion that could be had on national television, which was a risk I had identified ahead of the programme. When Savita was mentioned, No supporters laughed and jeered.

As Claire Byrne walked through the audience with the roving mic, it became clear that there had been some kind of mix-up. I was told later that No campaigners had pretended to be Yes supporters when applying for tickets, and so, when Claire Byrne approached a speaker, expecting him or her in that particular seat to be in favour of repeal, she found a No voter there instead. Her control of the situation quickly slipped away. It was like a bad episode of *The Jeremy Kyle Show* or, as I was to tell Pat Kenny on Newstalk the next morning, like something straight out of 'the Trump playbook'.

Worst of all, and totally inexcusably, not one parent from TFMR was asked to speak, even though they had been specifically invited and told they would have an opportunity to tell their stories. On the panel we could hear No supporters in the audience hissing and jeering the TFMR parents with taunts of 'murderers', but this was inaudible to the TV audience at home. There was no attempt by the RTÉ team to tell them to stop. Some Yes supporters felt physically intimidated.

John Monaghan reached a low point when he suggested my knowledge of fetal development was deficient, claiming, ludicrously, that there was no fetal development after twelve weeks and that if I didn't know that I needed to 'go back to school'. More cheering and hollering. I wondered what people thought goes on in the womb in the twenty-eight additional weeks before full term.

Mary Lou and Orla remained calm, with Mary Lou drawing on her considerable political experience. In the dressing room afterwards, however, she said she had never experienced anything like it. Never having been subjected to that level of vitriol and abuse before, I was definitely shaken by the experience. Claire Byrne also appeared shaken, and left the building almost immediately after the show. There were no sociable drinks in the Green Room.

18.   The end of the Eighth

In the cold light of day the morning after the *Claire Byrne Live* debate, there was rueful admission in the Together for Yes HQ that it had been right to fear the show would turn into a circus. The media were chalking it up as a win for the No campaign. It looked like taking the risk of sending me on had backfired.

However, I disagreed with the media take. It is a truism in sport that the losing team plays the man and not the ball, and clearly a key objective that evening had been to 'take Boylan out'. In trying to achieve this, the No side had overplayed their hand. It was telling that on that Tuesday huge numbers of new volunteers came on board the Together for Yes campaign around the country. And Mary Brosnan, director of midwifery at Holles Street and a long-standing and valued colleague, was so incensed by how I had been treated that she came into the Together for Yes HQ to make a video in support of repeal. It had over 100,000 views on various channels.

RTÉ received nearly 1,300 complaints, of which more than 90 per cent said that the Yes side had been badly treated. I think the conduct of the No side clarified to undecided voters the real alternatives in the referendum, exposed the viciousness of the No campaign and raised questions about what the No campaign was presenting as fact.

Still, there was much to be concerned about. Of all of the panellists, Maria Steen had had the most assured performance, even if it was as a consequence of seriously misrepresenting the proposed legislation. The Together for Yes team were worried that she had gained a credibility she had not previously enjoyed.

The greater fear, exacerbated by the dirty tricks of the leaked letter on the morning of the show, was that I was becoming the story. Already the No side's strategy of attacking me was becoming more intense by the day. I had been warned that serious pressure would be put on me, and so it proved. After Facebook's announcement the previous week that it would no longer be running referendum ads, abuse on social media had accelerated significantly. It was amusing to look at Twitter to see how much I was disliked in such places as Missouri, Alabama and Texas. Supporters of the National Rifle Association and President Trump seemed to be taking a keen interest in our referendum and did not like me very much. Some Irish No voters jumped in with enthusiasm, apparently not caring about the law on defamation or basic standards of decency. There was attention from Moscow, too. Clearly I was being targeted by troll farms in the US and possibly Russia. (Curiously, around 10 p.m. on the night before the referendum vote, most of the trolls went away. That was close of business US East Coast Time. The timing suggested that a contract had come to an end.)

However much I appreciated the Taoiseach's words in the Dáil the day after *Claire Byrne Live*, when he criticized the attempt to personalize the campaign around me, his intervention confirmed that there was a danger that I was becoming a distraction. So it was decided that, apart from a commitment in Waterford later in the week, I would be held back for one of the last major media events, the final RTÉ *Six One News* of the campaign. I called it going into 'stealth mode', and a blissful peace descended for a few days.

On the Friday evening a week before the vote, we went to Waterford for a public meeting organized by Minister of State John Halligan. He had quite an operation in the city, and his team were welcoming and enthusiastic. About 300 people attended including No voters, with one of whom, a local GP, I had a very civilized exchange. Any anxiety among local supporters that might have followed the *Claire Byrne Live* debacle had dissipated by then, and they were buoyed by the large attendance. Tara Flynn spoke movingly and with impact about her personal story, as did Claire Cullen Delsol of TFMR. Claire was in an advanced stage of pregnancy at that point, and her energy and commitment were admirable.

The next morning, freed temporarily from the campaign, Jane and I drove to Dungarvan and spent a peaceful hour looking at the war memorial and visiting the castle. We went on to Cappoquin House, where the early summer garden was magnificent. We were the only visitors, and Sir Charles Keane, the owner, came over to say hello. On seeing Jane's Together for Yes badge, he said, 'I approve!' He invited us in to look around the house and told us the history of the house and of his family. It was a magical interlude.

From there we went to the famous Barron's Bakery in the village for lunch. As we collected our sandwiches, we were told that 'We are all Yes voters around here.' Straws in the wind, perhaps, but we were being welcomed everywhere with smiles.

At the beginning of the final week of the campaign, Savita Halappanavar's father made a moving intervention, calling for a Yes vote.

My daughter, she lost her life because of this abortion law, because of the diagnosis, and she could not have an abortion. She died . . . I strongly feel that the younger daughters of Ireland should not have the fate of Savita. I hope the people of Ireland will remember the fate of our daughter Savita on the day of the referendum and vote Yes, so that what happened to us won't happen to any families. And by the doing this you will be paying a great debt to the departed soul.

It was a timely reminder of the tragedy of Savita's death, and how that devastating event had helped to galvanize the campaign for change.

Maria Steen's apparent triumph in the *Claire Byrne Live* debate had interesting consequences. Word on the grapevine was that relations between the two No campaigns – Save The 8th and Love Both – were deteriorating. Between them they had fewer volunteers than the Yes side and were getting tired and stretched. Egos were also starting to dominate. Buoyed by her *Claire Byrne Live* appearance, Maria Steen believed she would be a strong performer in further media events, and this resulted in Cora Sherlock being marginalized.

In the final week the No campaign imploded. A huge chink emerged in their central argument when they started hinting that something could be done for fetal abnormalities without repeal. Not only was this untrue, but the shift in position came too late, and, crucially, it undermined their core message that there were no problems with the Eighth and that termination was always wrong. Also, they couldn't find enough doctors to present their case. In the last few days of the campaign BBC Northern Ireland asked me to take part in a debate. I made it clear I would debate only with another doctor. The No side put up John McGuirk, so I declined to take part.

The decision to ask Minister Simon Harris to speak on the *Prime Time* debate on 22 May – three days out from polling – proved inspired. Mary Higgins was due to appear with him. Last minute chaos in the No campaign meant Peadar Tóibín of Sinn Féin was the only agreed speaker for their side. Behind the scenes, as the debate approached, apparently Maria Steen was insisting that she appear as the second panellist. Weeks before, however, RTÉ News and Current Affairs had made it clear that it required different panellists for its two televised debates.* Cora Sherlock was reluctantly put forward. But John McGuirk claimed that the No side heard only late in the day that an obstetrician was appearing on the Yes side. Because of that, he said, they wanted to replace Cora Sherlock with Maria Steen (though, like Sherlock, she was a lawyer, not an obstetrician; indeed, one of the few moments of light relief after *Claire Byrne Live* was that Steen's imperious declaration 'I'm the only lawyer on the panel' became a running joke on the Yes side). At the last moment Cora Sherlock was withdrawn in an attempt to bounce RTÉ into accepting Maria, but they held firm. So the debate was a head-to-head between Harris and Tóibín, with Mary Higgins taking a seat in the audience.

Peadar Tóibín is a good debater, but Simon Harris proved superb on the evening. When it was put to Minister Harris that termination was not a good option for a woman, as she might 'get over' the trauma of rape, he responded: 'Isn't there a better chance that the woman will make an informed decision of what's best for her and her family by being able to talk to her own doctor in her own country, rather than going to a strange land?' He noted that 'Women in this country are not going around *demanding* abortions, they're in crisis.' A repugnant feature of the No campaign's often graphic posters had been the absence of women from them. They were merely silhouettes or headless torsos, but Harris put women firmly to the fore in the debate, telling Tóibín that 'The greatest protector of a pregnancy is a mother, it's a woman, and I trust women to protect their pregnancies and you constantly don't trust them.'

The next night Pat Kenny moderated the TV3 debate. For the No side, Maria Steen and Senator Rónán Mullen; for Yes, Minister Regina Doherty and Colm O'Gorman of Amnesty International.

---

* *The Late Show* debate was outside the remit of the News and Current Affairs team, hence my appearance on it and subsequently on *Claire Byrne Live*.

I thought that putting Senator Mullen forward was a mistake, given that the No campaign needed to appeal to the undecided rather than their core vote, and he was not a man to appeal to the middle ground. In the studio that night there was a negative reaction to his claim that 'Mental health has no health base', as there was to him telling a young woman who told her story of having a termination that she deserved love and respect 'no matter what you've done'. Social media judged his comment as patronizing and unfeeling.

Maria Steen did better in trying to appeal to middle ground voters in continuing the pivot that the No side had been attempting in the previous few days: hinting that somehow the 'hard cases' could be dealt with without repeal. It was too little, too late and got little traction. Regina Doherty countered the point effectively, calling it a 'stunt' and reminding viewers that in recent years anti-abortion campaigners had vehemently and consistently opposed any attempts to liberalize abortion, including the Protection of Life During Pregnancy Act.

My last appearance for Together for Yes, on Wednesday, 23 May, saw Jane and me on the road to Donegal for the third time in nine weeks. On the drive up, I felt the weight of responsibility. There had been extensive preparation at HQ over the previous two days. As ever I had been impressed by the strategic nous of the communications experts. The importance of doing a good job for the campaign was clear. As we drove around the M50, Jane played Eamon Dunphy's podcast interview with conservative journalist John Waters on a continuous loop to relieve the tension. Dunphy's attempt to probe Waters' thinking about when life began provoked a furious reaction, and thirteen minutes into the interview he stormed out of the studio, shouting 'You're a bollocks, you're a fucking bollocks' at a bewildered and protesting Eamon. We wept laughing.

As we drove north, Jane stood in for *Six One* presenter Keelin Shanley and put possible questions to me. After a few minutes she stopped me, alarmed. She was not hearing my voice, she said. We carried on. She stopped me again. I was overthinking the interview. I was too anxious to stick to a script that, while it made the points eloquently, didn't sound like I had written it. Somewhere beyond Enniskillen, she said my voice was coming through again. She closed her notes, and we put on BBC Radio 4, where there was no referendum coverage.

On a beautiful sunny evening in the grounds of Donegal Castle, I waited to be interviewed for the last *Six One News* before the broadcast moratorium. The chaos in the No campaign was such that we were not sure who would be representing them. As it turned out, Niamh Uí Bhriain appeared. We had little conversation. I guess we were both battle-weary by then. Certainly, any enthusiasm I had for attempting a civilized engagement had disappeared.

I tried to make my last message as simple as possible: *It's okay to vote Yes on Friday. You will not be voting to introduce abortion to Ireland because it is already here, given the online availability of abortion pills. You will be voting Yes to looking after the women of Ireland in crisis pregnancies with compassion in the future.*

It is said that in referenda the majority of people only focus fully in the last few days. I had been confident of a Yes vote throughout the campaign. Over the course of my forty years in practice, and especially in more recent years, women around the country, many but not all of them former patients, had told me to continue to speak out. They were fed up with the interference of Church and state in their lives and wanted to change things for the better for their younger sisters.

The moratorium began at 2 p.m. on Thursday, 24 May. The campaign was over. It was up to the people now.

Jane and I decided to treat ourselves to a night in a hotel in town that evening. One of our boys was having a post-exam party at home, which was a further incentive. Before dinner we walked through the centre of Dublin. It was a beautiful early summer's evening. There seemed to be rivers of people wearing Yes badges. We stopped for a glass of wine in the Bull and Castle pub near Dublin Castle. When I went to pay, the manager said the drinks were on the house as a way of saying thank you. It was a touching gesture of support.

Along Essex Street in Temple Bar we came across the Together for Yes merchandise shop, which was crowded. A young woman outside the shop handed me a campaign leaflet with my photograph on it and inquired if I had decided on my vote yet. Then she looked at me properly, and we both burst out laughing.

There was an extraordinary buzz in the air. We were continually stopped by people wanting to chat, take selfies and hug. On Molesworth Street, we stopped outside Buswells Hotel and looked at Leinster House, agreeing that we had developed an increased respect for politicians of all parties over the course of the campaign, and in the months leading up to it. Many of them had struggled with the difficult issues raised by the referendum, but they had educated themselves, challenged long-held views and ultimately put women first.

After a peaceful breakfast at the hotel next morning with no referendum talk, we made our way to the Luas to go home to Ranelagh to vote, passing a Together for Yes stall at the top of Grafton Street. We had met one of the young volunteers on numerous occasions around the country over the past few weeks. She introduced us to her mother, and we told her she should be very proud of her daughter. Then we carried on home to vote.

There was a steady stream of voters making their way to our local polling station in the church hall. There seemed to be a good turnout, which I found reassuring. It was somewhat surreal to think that this might well be the end of a long journey to repeal the Eighth Amendment.

At 10 p.m. that night I was already asleep when Jane came upstairs to tell me that the *Irish Times* exit poll was showing an overwhelming majority for repeal. The RTÉ polls an hour and a half later confirmed the likely outcome. The relief was immense.

On Saturday morning we decided to go to the count centre at the RDS. On the way, I got a phone call asking when I was arriving, as some media wanted to talk to me. Could I phone when I was ten minutes away?

Nothing could have prepared me for the reception as I walked into the Simmonscourt Pavilion. A horde of reporters holding microphones, mobile phones, notebooks and television cameras bore down on me. I told them that it was a victory for the women of Ireland and that my experience over the years in talking to women, particularly older women, was that they were ready for this change, and it wasn't just the issue of abortion, it was the way women had been treated by this state over the years.

'We all know the litany of abuse that women and children have suffered,' I said, 'so I think it was part of the sequence of redress for all of the wrongs over the years.'

Thus began one of the most extraordinary days of my life. After spending around an hour in the counting centre, Jane and I went to the Intercontinental Hotel, where the Together for Yes campaigners were gathering. A large ballroom was packed, and the campaign team were coming to the microphone for short speeches. I was called forward; I thanked everyone for their support; I said that, although I had retired from clinical practice, and although many of my colleagues who also had retired went on to do further studies, I wouldn't be going 'back to school'. That got a laugh.

Next stop was the RTÉ studios for a results programme hosted by Bryan Dobson. There were four panellists, including Deputy Mattie McGrath, who was sitting beside me. During a break, I asked him why he had accused me of lying on *Claire Byrne Live*. He said he had not called me a liar, but that I had been 'peddling lies'. I decided not to follow him down that particular rabbit hole.

We went on to Dublin Castle, where there was a large crowd in front of the stage in the courtyard. The mood was emotional and joyous. It was an odd experience to hear the crowd cheering and calling my name. The stage was jammed with people who had been campaigning against the Eighth, some for decades. The atmosphere was one of immense relief. Over and over, women commented that they felt like equal citizens in their own country for the first time.

The media did a good job in an obstacle course of cables, tripods and lights. I was interviewed by Kay Burley of Sky News, a surreal experience, but I got the impression that the veteran journalist was startled by events, not fully understanding the significance of the vote in the context of the historical treatment of women in Ireland.

Some later criticized the air of celebration that pervaded the Castle yard that Saturday. In my opinion, celebration was justified. The outcome of the referendum represented a rejection of the hypocrisy in our Constitution that had harmed women for decades. In voting to repeal the Eighth Amendment, we had taken one more critical step in Ireland's journey to becoming a true republic. It signalled both our maturity and our compassion. The Taoiseach encapsulated it well when he spoke later:

Today, we as a people have spoken. And we say that we trust women and we respect women and their decisions. For me it is also the day when we said No More. No more doctors telling their patients there is nothing that can be done for them in their own country. No more lonely journeys across the Irish Sea. No more stigma. The veil of secrecy is lifted. No more isolation. The burden of shame is gone.

We left the Castle for a pub across the way with Deirdre Duffy, a group from Together for Yes and some politicians from different parties who had been prominent in the campaign. Everyone had been moved by the atmosphere in the Castle. Later Jane and I walked, or attempted to walk, along Dame Lane with Senator Ivana Bacik. Crowds from the restaurants and pubs had spilled on to the street on the warm May night, and the atmosphere was incredible. Nearly thirty years earlier, when Ivana was president of the students' union in Trinity, anti-abortion activists had attempted to have her imprisoned for providing abortion information in the students' union handbook, and as a Labour Party politician she had been a strong campaigner against the Eighth. People were queuing up to thank her for all she had done. Again, every few steps there were handshakes, hugs and selfies. We took a photo with a group of lawyers wearing T-shirts bearing the legend 'I'm the only lawyer on the panel'. They promised to send me one and they were true to their word.

Eventually, Jane and I made it to the far end of Trinity Street. It had taken over an hour to walk the short distance. We got a taxi and, exhausted and drained, went home to sleep.

19.   And now, the practicalities

On 18 September President Higgins signed the Thirty-sixth Amendment into law. And so the way was clear for the government to work towards the 1 January deadline it had set itself for introducing an abortion service. Coordination would be the key to making sure that the new service integrated smoothly into the overall health service. However, at the Oireachtas Committee hearing on 17 September, it had been apparent that there had been little coordination to date. Since my term as chair of the Institute was ending on 28 September and I would have more free time, I phoned Simon Harris and suggested that someone needed to drive the project and coordinate the different elements, and if he thought it might be useful, I was available. The Minister agreed.

The initial plan was that I would be appointed as clinical adviser to the Minister, but this ruffled some feathers in the Department of Health, so it was agreed I would be attached to the HSE's National Women and Infants Health Programme (NWIHP), led by Kilian McGrane. It didn't much matter to me what my title was, as long as the job got done. The Minister took care to announce my appointment himself, which made it clear to all that I had his imprimatur.

The next three months were among the busiest of my professional life as, almost immediately, it became apparent that my role would be a combination of adviser, mediator and troubleshooter, operating within a process that involved multiple moving parts. When I look back at my diary for the period, I see that I attended eighty-three meetings, dialled into daily conference calls, and visited most of the maternity hospitals or maternity units around the country.

Immediately after my appointment, on 2 October, the Minister convened a meeting with all relevant groups, including Dr Tony Holohan, the Department of Health's Chief Medical Officer, Kilian McGrane and Dr Peter McKenna of the NWIHP, Cliona Murphy from the Institute, Mary Favier and John O'Brien from the Irish College of General Practitioners (ICGP), Dr Suzanne Crowe and Bill Prasifka from the Medical Council, Mike Thompson and Trish

Horgan from the Southern Taskgroup on Abortion and Reproductive Topics (START), an umbrella group of obstetricians and gynaecologists and GPs from Cork and the South-West, Maeve Taylor and Dr Caitriona Henchion from the Irish Family Planning Association (IFPA), Alison Begas and Dr Shirley McQuaid from the Dublin Well Woman Centre, and representatives from the HSE and Department of Health.

Those present were enthusiastic about getting the service up and running, but agreed that an immense amount of work was needed to be ready for 1 January. The main concerns were about resourcing, dealing with conscientious objection and the need for clinical guidelines.

In addition, the community doctors (GPs and doctors attached to the family planning clinics) had concerns about liability insurance, how the service would be funded, education and guidelines, access to ultrasound for dating a pregnancy and to blood testing to check for rhesus negativity, the availability of abortion pills in the community, the clinical pathway into a hospital in the event of complication or if the pregnancy was further advanced than nine weeks, follow-up after a termination, the unavailability of free contraception. The GPs emphasized the looming crisis in general practice due to the number of retirements coming down the tracks and the difficulties of retaining staff due to poor working conditions. GPs had been hit hard by the cuts arising from the financial crisis a decade earlier, and the recent Budget had imposed another 100,000 Medical Card patients on them.

Apart from the practical issues, I was conscious that the new service would be a huge cultural change in Irish medical practice. I had observed that, while there may have been enthusiasm for repeal of the Eighth among many obstetricians, what that would mean, in practice, particularly in the nine-to-twelve weeks category, presented challenges for some of them. This was understandable, as repeal was an abstract concept, whereas performing a termination was a concrete action. I think this partly explains some colleagues' public reticence during the campaign. As I was retired from clinical practice, this was not a dilemma that I had to face so I had a lot of sympathy for them.

There are nuances and complexities in every area of life, and this is especially true with abortion, where deep philosophical and moral arguments can arise. There are many things that deter doctors from providing abortions. Abortion might be personally objectionable or contrary to their religious beliefs. They might have to face the memory of their own previous abortion experience, or worry about their reputation with colleagues. Perhaps significant people in their lives oppose abortion, or they are concerned about their personal safety and fear harassment or violence by those opposed to abortion. Doctors might well be comfortable with one woman's abortion decision, but challenged by the circumstances surrounding another – for example, some might be willing to perform a termination on a fifteen-year-old who is pregnant, having been raped, but not on a 34-year-old woman pregnant after a one-night stand.

It is only natural that, in spite of efforts to be objective, doctors hold personal values that influence how they respond to patients. It is also the case that one's values may change in response to life experiences and to encounters with patients and colleagues. While my engagement with the cases of Savita Halappanavar, Miss P and Ms Y had had a profound influence on my views about the harm caused by the Eighth Amendment, other doctors had not had the same exposure. Also, while the harmful and sometimes fatal consequences when abortion is illegal or otherwise inaccessible is well documented, in Ireland doctors working in hospitals had not been exposed to the awful effects of illegal abortion, because of the availability of abortion in the UK and Europe.

With all of this in mind, at the Institute we felt that a programme of 'values clarification education' was essential in the context of introducing an abortion service, as its success would be dependent on the cooperation of doctors. The purpose of values clarification education is to help doctors, midwives and other healthcare professionals in examining and understanding their personal beliefs about abortion so that they are better able to care for women considering terminations. It emphasizes the difficulty with comparing one patient's situation with another's. Cliona Murphy and Maeve Eogan of the Rotunda arranged for the World Health Organization to provide the first educational sessions, with local doctors and midwives trained to spearhead the education into the future. Feedback shows that those who took part in the initial sessions found them very useful, and some changed their minds in favour of participating in the service.

★

When it came to the practical introduction of abortion services, there was a long list of issues to be sorted before they could commence. Some difficulties were anticipated; some only arose as the planning process got under way. This was against a backdrop of constant noise from the media, politicians and doctors expressing doubt that the 1 January deadline would – or should – be met. Inevitably, given human nature, there seemed to be more focus on raising problems than providing solutions. My approach was to deal with problems as they arose and work through them step by step. As a doctor, I had no political capital invested in meeting the January deadline, but I thought it only right that the referendum result should be implemented as soon as was practicable. Women had waited long enough, and we had been talking for long enough. In the absence of a deadline, matters could drift.

Abortion services were to be provided in three categories: up to nine weeks in the community; nine to twelve weeks in hospitals; over twelve weeks in hospitals for fatal fetal abnormalities and in cases where there was a substantial risk to the life or health of a woman. The first task was to establish how the service would be provided for each category and what resources would be needed. I decided to approach it from the woman's perspective, starting with the moment she found out she was pregnant and, for whatever reason, decided she could not continue with the pregnancy.

Already the HSE had decided that a website and 24-hour telephone helpline should be set up as the first point of contact for a woman seeking information or assistance, and had set about creating what became the My Options website and helpline. The team putting it together paid a lot of attention to detail. For instance, when it came to the use of language, they held focus groups with members of the public to help ensure the language on the site was user-friendly and non-technical. Participants were asked if it was better to use 'termination of pregnancy', which is the medical term, or 'abortion'. Abortion was preferred. Similarly, 'unplanned pregnancy' was preferred to 'crisis pregnancy'. When it went live on 20 December, the My Options site gave detailed information, in easily understood language, on all the options in the case of an unplanned pregnancy. Following the introduction of abortion services on 1 January there were over 600,000 page views and 170,000 visits to the website by the end of May 2019. Its success is a credit to the hard work of the team that developed it.

The helpline, meanwhile, is staffed by trained nurses from One Family, an organization with considerable experience in crisis pregnancy counselling. It is accessed through the My Options website and operates twenty-four hours a day, seven days a week. There are two elements to it. First, information is provided on next steps depending on an individual woman's circumstances, for example the name of a nearby GP who provides the service. An average of fifty-eight calls a day were received in January, falling to thirty-one by April, indicating an element of pent-up demand in December 2018, as women waited for the service to start in the New Year. Second, if a woman is experiencing complications such as bleeding, a nurse is available to give advice. This service received an average of ten calls a day in the first four months, with an average wait time of thirteen seconds before the phone was answered. By any yardstick this is an impressive performance.

Moving on to the next stage – women going to their GPs for terminations – based on guesstimates of Irish women going abroad for terminations or accessing abortion pills online, the HSE estimated that around 10,000 terminations would be performed each year in the under-twelve-weeks category. Of that figure it was thought that at least 80 per cent – or 8,000 terminations – would be before nine weeks and so would be performed by GPs. The 10,000 figure was also based on the experience of Scotland and Norway, two neighbouring countries with populations similar to Ireland in size and distribution, with the figures adjusted for the Irish population. This was a higher figure than that of women giving Irish addresses when travelling to the UK or accessing pills online. However, given the stigma and illegality of the past, those figures had probably not captured the full picture. HSE planners took the view that it was better to overestimate than underestimate the numbers of women who might use the service.

In the October 2018 Budget, €12 million was allocated to the roll-out of the new abortion service, with Minister Harris commenting that 'This is not something that can in any way be short-changed.' That €12 million did not include costs for ancillary recommendations such as free contraception. These would be funded by the 'additional services' provision in the Budget that would be contingent upon the negotiations of the new GPs' contract.

At the end of October the Minister told me he would be able to offer a generous package for the community service, and a few weeks later it was announced that doctors who accepted the new contract would receive a total fee of €450 covering three visits – made up of a payment of €150 to cover the initial consultation with the patient and a further €300 for carrying out the termination procedure and the delivery of aftercare.

By 1 December 121 GPs had signed the contract, with around 200 signed up when services commenced in January. Inevitably perhaps, the focus turned to the number of GPs who had not signed, with negative commentary that the modest number contracted somehow represented failure.

A number of GPs were vehemently opposed to the introduction of the service despite the referendum result. At an EGM of the ICGP on 2 December 2018, fifty of around 300 GPs present staged a disruptive and noisy walkout after they failed to get a number of motions from the floor accepted. Considerable abuse was levelled at Fintan Foy, the CEO, but he kept his cool and sense of purpose.

At the time of writing (August 2019), around 325 GPs provide the service. If, for the sake of argument, the anticipated 8,000 terminations were divided equally among them, this would give a workload of twenty-four terminations per doctor per year. As I write, however, it looks like the number of terminations annually may be closer to 5,000, which would mean an average of twelve cases for each GP every year – or one a month. Clearly, therefore, there is ample GP provision.

There remain some areas with poorer coverage than others, though as time goes on it is improving. At the beginning of 2019 there was concern that some women would have to travel outside their county in order to see a doctor. This is, however, a massive improvement on having to leave the country. Indeed, for reasons of confidentiality some women may prefer not to attend their local GP, but to travel to a nearby town or city.

A more significant potential problem for GPs than additional workload was to do with liability insurance. GPs insure themselves with either the Medical Protection Society (MPS) in the UK or Medisec, an Irish company underwritten by Allianz. The MPS had no difficulty with indemnity, but a potential difficulty for the implementation deadline arose when, fearing high Irish legal claims, it appeared that Medisec was reluctant to provide cover. Switching between companies was not all that simple, so this could be a challenge for Medisec clients. However, after some discussion, Medisec agreed to provide indemnity on the quite reasonable condition that GPs had the necessary training.

One of the biggest headaches for the community service was the provision of ultrasound. GPs would need rapid access to scanning if there was any doubt about dates, or if there was concern that a pregnancy might be ectopic (outside the womb). However, almost no GPs had ultrasound scanners, and maternity hospitals and maternity units had little or no spare capacity.

Discussions were started with Affidea, a private company that provides diagnostic imaging in sixteen countries around Europe, and that was already performing over 10,000 ultrasound scans, MRIs and CT scans for the HSE every year. Contracting Affidea seemed an ideal solution.

Since Affidea did not provide pregnancy scanning as part of its existing service, it did not employ the necessary specially trained ultrasonographers.* This did not seem like it should be a problem – in maternity hospitals, scans are performed by trained midwives who can explain the findings to patients immediately without waiting – perhaps several days – for a doctor to deliver results. These scans are relatively straightforward: all that is required is confirmation that the pregnancy is in the uterus, is ongoing and how far advanced it is, and is not a twin pregnancy. Affidea suggested that it would employ midwife sonographers to solve the problem.

All seemed well until it emerged that HSE requirements about ultrasonography were particularly onerous. So, while one arm of the HSE – the one trying to get the abortion service off the ground – was happy for Affidea to employ midwives, another arm – the one charged with professional standards – was insisting that the ultrasonographers needed a full radiology degree. This had the potential to delay implementation by many months.

In my role as troubleshooter I stepped in and explained why it was acceptable to employ appropriately trained midwives. I met complete refusal. I tried again – UCD's B.Sc. course in ultrasonography takes

---

* Ultrasonographers are specialists in performing ultrasound scans.

four years, but UCD also provides a six-month professional certificate in early pregnancy ultrasound qualification, so I suggested this as a solution. This was also refused. So inflexible was the response to all suggestions that I wondered if it was ideologically driven. It was one of the worst moments of the implementation project.

In the end Affidea was able to locate enough ultrasonographers and radiologists with sufficient experience of early pregnancy scanning to provide a limited service in a few locations around the country. It may not have been ideal, but it solved a major problem.

Once the scans were done, they had to be reviewed and signed off by a doctor. The reports had then to be provided in a timely fashion to the GPs and family planning clinics that were referring women for scans, because of the need to meet the nine weeks deadline for termination in the community. It became clear at the end of November that there would be a problem with reporting the scans, as Affidea didn't have anyone on staff regularly reporting on early pregnancy scans. One of their consultants had done so some years previously but felt he was a bit rusty, so I agreed to review the scans and do the reports myself for the first two months following the introduction of the service. It had the benefit of giving me daily insight into how the service was working and allowed me to assess the quality of the scans being performed. I was impressed by the high quality and I detected no errors in the two months.

As time went on, it was interesting to note that the average gestation at which women were presenting for scans declined progressively, so that by February 2019 almost 90 per cent were less than nine weeks pregnant at the time of presentation to their GP or family planning clinic. I have been reliably informed that that figure has remained constant to the time of writing in August 2019. This means of course that a higher number of terminations than anticipated are taking place in the community, putting us in line with Norway and Scotland (as I had said we would be throughout the referendum campaign).

The HSE had contracted Affidea on the assumption that there might be a requirement for 10,000 scans per year (a very generous estimate, given that the HSE expected about 8,000 abortions to be community-based and a minority of women presenting to GPs would require an ultrasound). However, based on the figures of approximately 120 per month for the first seven months of the service, it looks like the requirement will be more like 1,500 per year.

Another area of concern for GPs was whether or not women having terminations who have rhesus negative blood would need an injection of Anti-D immunoglobulin. Approximately 15 per cent of women living in Ireland have rhesus negative blood. A problem arises when fetal blood is rhesus positive and enters the mother's bloodstream, because there is a risk of her developing antibodies that might cause problems in future pregnancies. This risk is minimized by administration of Anti-D. Although the risk in early pregnancy is minimal, current RCOG guidelines recommend the administration of Anti-D to all rhesus negative women who have terminations at more than seven weeks gestation.

A protocol for Ireland needed to be worked out, but opinion among colleagues was divided. A possible downside of the administration of Anti-D is that it is a natural blood product, so there is a possibility of contamination. On the other hand, there was a fear that if Anti-D was not administered, a woman might go on to develop antibodies in later pregnancy. As this is Ireland, I am quite sure that fear of litigation was in the minds of some colleagues.

Eventually in early December, after much discussion, the Institute and the ICGP sought consultant haematologist input. Our haematology colleagues were anxious to avert any risk of an issue like the hepatitis C problem of the 1990s* and took a cautious line. In the end it was agreed to proceed according to current RCOG guidelines, although these may change at a later date.

The medications used in medical terminations are mifepristone, followed by misoprostol. Mifepristone blocks the production of progesterone, the hormone that supports the pregnancy before the placenta is developed. The medication was first approved for use in France in 1998, but had never been licensed in Ireland. This created

---

* In the mid 90s it emerged that Anti-D created from blood provided by donors suffering from hepatitis C had been given to 1,200 Irish women. It cost many of these women their health and even their lives, and the cost to the state in compensation and costs is estimated to be over €1 billion.

no difficulties and it was authorized for use on 30 November, pending the successful passage of the legislation.

Misoprostol (which makes the uterus contract) was already licensed for treatment of stomach ulcers under the trade name of Cytotec and is used extensively off-licence in maternity hospitals for the treatment of miscarriage.* Given Ireland's highly litigious culture, the GPs feared legal action if there were problems. A series of meetings with the ICGP and the Health Products Regulatory Authority (HPRA) was needed to provide the reassurance the GPs needed.

However, we were by no means out of the woods on this just yet. The pharmaceutical firm Nordic, which was due to provide the mifepristone, had a number of concerns that threatened to derail the supply. On 17 December, just two weeks before the service was due to start, the firm's medical director came from Paris to join her two Dublin-based colleagues for a crisis meeting with Dr Tony Holohan, the Chief Medical Officer, Geraldine Luddy, a senior official in the Department of Health, Kate Mulvenna from the HSE and myself.

One of Nordic's concerns was that the tablets would be supplied to unknown pharmacies and then transferred onwards to doctors unknown to them. We were able to reassure them that only pharmacies approved by the HSE would be supplied with the tablets and only doctors who had signed the contract would be eligible to receive them.

However, the Nordic team's main source of anxiety was about dosage. When Nordic developed mifepristone in the 1990s the recommended dosage based on research at that time was 600mg. Regulatory approval to market the medication was granted on that basis, and so the product information leaflet that accompanies every medication states this as the dosage. In the meantime, research around the world has shown conclusively that a lower dose of 200mg is just as effective, and has fewer side effects. This is now the recommended dosage in every country with legal medical termination of pregnancy services. Even in the United States, possibly the most litigious nation on earth, the American College of Obstetricians and Gynecologists (ACOG) recommends the 200mg dosage (despite the higher dose being what is officially approved).

---

* Off-licence means use for a purpose other than what the licence was granted for. This is not unusual in the practice of medicine.

Nordic has not updated the dosage information: to do so would require repeating the arduous and expensive licence application process, which would make no sense, particularly as the medication is now off-patent. Nordic is the only manufacturer of mifepristone.

The plan was that Irish guidelines would mirror those of the RCOG, the ACOG and the professional bodies of other countries around the world. However, given our high level of medical litigation, Nordic became very nervous about this. It seemed to me that they were particularly concerned about liability if, for example, there was a case of an unsuccessful termination and an ongoing pregnancy.

I think the publicity surrounding the implementation process also made them anxious and cautious. There had been consistently negative media coverage and some rather over-the-top opinion pieces written by doctors suggesting that plans for the new service were being rushed through with no regard for safety, best practice or quality of care. In an *Irish Times* opinion piece ten days before the Nordic meeting, the Coombe's Chris Fitzpatrick had said that it was 'dangerously unrealistic [to implement] a new termination of pregnancy service, which, if rushed into operation on January 1 as scheduled, will pose a serious threat to the health and wellbeing of women'.

He also criticized me, saying, '[M]eanwhile, Dr Boylan tells us that abortion will be available "in some form" in all nineteen maternity units in January and seeks to reassure the public that "the pieces are falling into place" while at the same time cautioning that "inevitably, there will be problems." This is not language that inspires confidence and Irish women deserve better.' Had he phoned me before writing the piece, I might have been able to ease his concerns. The pieces were in fact falling into place one by one at that stage.

A couple of days later Keelin O'Donoghue wrote in the *Sunday Business Post* that '[T]he reality is that we will not be able to introduce a safe high-quality or accessible service in January 2019.' She added that '[P]oliticians and managers currently congratulating themselves on passing legislation and providing a "woman-centred" termination of pregnancy service on January 1 display little interest in, or understanding of, the real complexities of working in maternity hospitals.'

These articles caused enormous irritation to the dozens of people working flat out for months on planning for the service, as the doctors' criticism was seen as long on rhetoric but short on facts or detail.

The stakes could scarcely have been higher, and the meeting with Nordic was tense. I asked if there had been a successful lawsuit anywhere in the world following use of the lower dosage. There had not. Yet there was no sign of the Nordic team changing its position as the meeting went on.

After a couple of hours, and with no compromise in the offing, the medical director indicated that she would return to Paris for consultation, and let us know the decision in a few days. This was alarming, given there were only fourteen days to go before the service was due to start, and Christmas was a week away. I thought it likely that from the distance of Paris it would be easy for the company simply to refuse to supply the medication. I asked her to reconsider and suggested we take a twenty-minute break to give everyone a breather.

When we returned to the room, we found that whatever conversation the Nordic team had had during our absence seemed to have resolved their anxieties, and they now agreed to supply the tablets, as long as it was made clear that the lower dose was not what the company recommended. This was a very reasonable suggestion. We agreed and suddenly the crisis was resolved.*

A final concern for the community doctors was that they – and their staff – might be subjected to harassment by demonstrators if it became known that they were providing an abortion service. GPs were no doubt mindful of the repugnant conduct of one particular anti-repeal group, which had displayed graphic images outside maternity hospitals during the referendum campaign as pregnant women and their children entered and left. This group, and others, had adopted aggressive tactics such as filming and recording passers-by. Such was the level of concern that some GPs began to remove identifying photos from their practice websites. The family planning clinics felt particularly vulnerable because it was obvious that they would be providing the service.

The Minister committed to drafting legislation to ensure that demonstrators could not come within a certain distance of doctors'

---

* In practice, the medication is supplied in a blister pack of three 200mg pills. A revised dosage label is attached to the outside of the box, and the GP cuts off one tablet to give to the patient.

premises, clinics or hospitals. At the time of writing the legislation has not yet passed, but should not be delayed, especially in light of demonstrations outside the National Maternity Hospital during the summer of 2019, when protestors placed small white coffins on the pavement outside the door of one of the antenatal clinics. As well as the small number of women attending the hospital for terminations, other women and families who are undergoing fertility treatment, or who have suffered miscarriage, still-birth or the death of a baby, are naturally distressed and shocked to see these coffins.

Ireland's abortion service differs from America's and the UK's, where stand-alone clinics are the norm. In Ireland the service is embedded into the healthcare system. It is impossible, therefore, for demonstrators to target individual women who might be going to their GP for, perhaps, a chest infection, to a family planning clinic for contraception, or into a maternity hospital for a regular antenatal appointment or because they are having a miscarriage.

Many GPs do not want to provide abortion, and that is their prerogative. Their patient demographics may be such that it makes little sense for them. Overall, however, in the implementation of the new abortion service, Irish GPs have demonstrated that they are practical, flexible and adept at finding solutions to problems as they arise.

20.   'How did we send these patients away before?'

From the beginning it was clear that the hospitals would present the greatest challenge when it came to implementing abortion services. Most doctors in Irish hospitals had never dealt with termination in early pregnancy before, and so anxiety about that change in medical practice, coupled with understandable frustration over infrastructure and resource issues, was going to make for difficult conversations.

In October and November, six months after my referendum odyssey around Ireland, I took to the road again, this time to visit the maternity hospitals and units around the country, so that I could meet as many of the consultant and midwifery staff as possible. There was a general willingness to provide the service, but – exactly as I had anticipated – staff had many concerns about introducing a new service when the existing infrastructure was already overstretched and creaking. It was clear that my first task was to listen to concerns and give the medical staff an opportunity to vent their feelings about their problems.

In particular, there was a lack of suitable space to hold clinics, a scarcity of inpatient beds and problems with access to operating theatres, which, in some hospitals, were either closed for some days during the week or simply not available to be used because of lack of staff or funding. Ultrasound services were overloaded. There were shortages of staff in every unit. Some gynaecology units that were integrated into general hospitals shared their wards with surgical patients, and all these units had long waiting lists for benign gynaecology procedures, with cancellations not uncommon in the winter months due to overcrowding in emergency departments and pressure from hospital management to reduce 'trolley counts' as much as possible to avoid negative media attention. Given all of these issues, teams in hospitals feared that the number of patients presenting would be beyond their ability to cope.

In Cork University Maternity Hospital they were concerned about additional numbers, given that they were still waiting for the commissioning of an operating theatre a decade after the new maternity hospital had been opened. As I mentioned earlier (see Chapter 12), this failure had led to unacceptably long gynaecological waiting lists. Disgracefully, that new operating theatre is still not functioning.

University Maternity Hospital in Limerick is configured in such a way as to provide access to the operating theatre through the corridor of the labour ward, a highly unsatisfactory situation both for women who have had miscarriages and for those having terminations. There was absolutely no prospect of gaining access to the general hospital in Limerick for surgical terminations, as it was completely overloaded. The hospital had submitted a plan to the HSE for a development that would address most of their concerns, but they had not received approval to proceed.

In University Hospital Galway, meanwhile, pressure on gynaecological services was such that one of the consultants had a three-year operating theatre waiting list. Letterkenny General Hospital had capacity issues, with an operating theatre there also awaiting commission. Conscientious objection was also an issue in Letterkenny, as it was in Cavan General Hospital, where, it was explained to me, some nurses refused to assist in the operating theatre even in cases of tubal ligation because of the nature of the procedure. In both hospitals staff assured me that they had no objections to treating patients for complications of terminations carried out in the community if that was required.

When I visited Our Lady of Lourdes Hospital, Drogheda, I found that there was concern about a possible influx of women coming from Northern Ireland, but otherwise, despite significant infrastructural problems, they were very willing to provide the service.

In Wexford General Hospital they had concerns about conscientious objection but intended to provide values clarification education. They were worried about bed shortages in winter months, and that one of three operating theatres was closed three days a week due to staff shortages.

My visits to the various units around the country were further evidence, if it was needed, that integration of maternity and gynaecology services into general hospitals is having a very negative effect on the ability of staff to give women the dignity and treatment they deserve.

The three Dublin maternity hospitals were always going to be key. They serve the most populous region of the country and are also tertiary referral centres, therefore dealing with the majority of fatal fetal abnormality cases. They are voluntary hospitals run by a master, not owned by the HSE or Catholic religious orders, so they have full autonomy in their operation. I met all three masters as soon as possible after taking up my advisory role at the beginning of October.

In the Rotunda, Fergal Malone had identified a space in the hospital suitable for conversion to an outpatient gynaecology centre and undertook to provide financial estimates to the HSE. He did not anticipate problems with conscientious objection.

In the Coombe, Sharon Sheehan outlined infrastructural deficits, particularly in the early pregnancy assessment unit. The Coombe had 3,000 patients on its gynaecology outpatient waiting list, and a nine-month waiting list for benign surgery. The master suggested that the building of a modular clinic for outpatient gynaecology on top of the existing modular colposcopy clinic would make a very satisfactory termination of pregnancy service possible. Her position, however, was that the Coombe would not be ready to provide the service on 1 January due to lack of guidelines, staff shortages and the infrastructural issues. There was obviously no prospect of recruiting additional staff or extending the modular unit by 1 January, but the guidelines had been in development for several months already and should be available, so I encouraged the master to submit plans in the meantime for the extension.

My jaw dropped, however, when I met Rhona Mahony and other staff at the National Maternity Hospital at the end of October. They said they would need no fewer than twenty-seven additional full-time staff members to provide termination of pregnancy services. They had other requests as well – for MRI funding and operating theatre space.

In order to illustrate how that level of additional staffing would not be required, I took them through the anticipated numbers they could expect. If around 35 per cent of the expected total 10,000 terminations annually took place in Dublin, that would give an annual figure of 3,500, or around 300 a month. Some 80 per cent of those were likely to be in the community, but even over-estimating, and working on a 60 per cent/40 per cent community-to-hospital ratio, the three Dublin hospitals would have no more than 120 cases a month between them, i.e., 40 a month, or 10 a week each, at most.★ Of those 10 per week, 5 were likely to be medical and 5 surgical. To put this in context, in 2016 there were 6,420 operative procedures at the NMH and approximately 16,700 women attended the gynae-cology/colposcopy service.

I advised Dr Mahony and her team that it would do their relation-ship with the Department of Health no good to submit a request for twenty-seven new staff members for a likely maximum extra work-load of ten patients each week.†

The possibility of doing surgical termination operating lists at weekends was considered in the Holles Street meeting. The NMH team pointed out that nurses would only get paid an extra €6 for working on a Saturday, and there was therefore unlikely to be great enthusiasm for this particular solution. This was understandable and another illustration of the difficulties in running a health service seven days a week, which some commentators simplistically suggest as a solution to waiting lists.

A couple of hours after my meeting in Holles Street concluded, the three masters wrote a joint letter to the Minister for Health, saying that they would not be ready by 1 January. I found this difficult to understand, since it had been clear within a couple of weeks of the referendum that the service was to start at the beginning of the New Year. Five months had passed since then and there were two months still to go. There were seven months available, in other words, to get organized.

In the Department of Health and the HSE there was a good deal of annoyance over this no-can-do attitude. The HSE was irritated because several months had passed since it had asked the masters to tell it what resources they needed, but nothing had been forth-coming. The Minister was also irritated, not only because the letter said that their hospitals wouldn't be ready in January but also because

---

★ As it turned out, once the service became established in 2019, the numbers were far fewer than feared, with the Dublin maternity hospitals seeing around five cases per week each.

† In February 2019 Holles Street advertised two new consultant positions – for an obstetrician/gynaecologist and an anaesthesiologist – to be funded from an HSE financial allocation for the provision of termination of pregnancy services.

the masters gave no indication as to when they would be ready. The tone was a little *take it or leave it*.

Having always been a strong advocate of the mastership system of management – where the master has the authority to direct resources, scarce though they may be, to whatever area of the hospital needs it most – I was particularly disappointed by the masters' letter. And, as both Rhona Mahony and Fergal Malone had been effective public advocates for repeal of the Eighth, I had difficulty in understanding their seeming tardiness.

Undaunted by this apparent set-back, the Minister and the various implementation groups continued to press ahead, and, as it transpired, both the NMH* and the Rotunda introduced the service from 1 January after all. The Coombe eventually caught up in early February.

A week after the Dublin masters' letter to Simon Harris, another problem arose when Keelin O'Donoghue in Cork and Peter McParland in Holles Street, together with twenty-two fetal medicine colleagues, also wrote to the Minister to say that they would not be ready on 1 January to provide terminations for fatal fetal abnormalities. Their chief concern appeared to be that they were, as they described it, 'unclear how structured services were to be implemented and who exactly bears responsibility for this in the extremely short proposed timeframe'.

To my mind, the answer was that they themselves were responsible for the provision of the service, considering that they were the leading fetal medicine specialists in the country, and it was up to the CEOs of the hospital groups to ensure that adequate staffing and facilities were in place. However, the group CEOs appeared not to be sufficiently engaged with the introduction of the service. To their credit, however, since the introduction of the service the fetal medicine specialists have provided excellent care to patients and are fully on board.

The letters of the masters and the fetal medicine consultants highlight two issues that need reflection by colleagues. First, the role of a senior medical consultant brings with it responsibility, and an obligation to provide leadership. Waiting for the HSE or Department is

---

* As it happened, the NMH's new master, Shane Higgins, started his term on 1 January 2019, too.

unlikely to be fruitful. Second, I would urge colleagues to think care-fully before signing round-robin letters that are sent to Ministers, newspapers or colleagues. Too often they are written in haste when feelings are high, and are reviewed with insufficient attention by doc-tors on their phones in the middle of busy clinics and ward rounds, or late at night after a long day in the hospital. A phone call or meeting to express concerns directly is more likely to be effective. It is probably a good idea to consider how one might feel seeing the letter in question on the front pages of the newspapers, as happens all too often. We might like to think that as highly trained people operating at senior levels we assess situations and take action based on entirely objective and rational grounds, but personality factors, personal feelings and stress come into play, too. Invariably, this makes arriving at a good outcome more frac-tious than it needs to be, as I have learned – sometimes because of having erred in this respect myself – over the years.

At a Department of Health meeting chaired by Simon Harris on 12 November, to which all stakeholders across the hospitals and the community were invited, there was understandable anxiety about the deadline. Sharon Sheehan said that the three masters did not feel they would be ready and asked, rather pointedly, who ultimately had responsibility for implementation.

Behind Sharon Sheehan's question was the valid concern that the medical profession would be blamed if the service was not successful. This reflected doctors' understandable anger at the underinvestment in maternity services over the years and the many tragedies that could be blamed, partly at least, on structural deficiencies as a con-sequence of underinvestment and dysfunctional governance. The Minister gave a direct answer: the National Women and Infants Health Programme would be responsible – in other words, the HSE.

In my view the correct answer is rather different – in medicine the buck stops with the doctor dealing with the patient. This is one of the features that makes medicine such a high-stakes but rewarding profes-sion. However, in order for doctors to be able to do their job, hospital management (i.e., the masters in the case of the Dublin maternity hos-pitals) is responsible for ensuring that the appropriate facilities are in place for the doctors; the HSE is responsible for ensuring that suffi-cient funds are provided to hospital management for appropriate staffing and facilities; the Department of Health is responsible for disbursing funds to the HSE; the Minister is responsible for ensuring enough funds are available from the Budget; and the Cabinet is responsible for the ultimate decisions on the allocation of funds to the different departments. There are many layers of responsibility.

There was a danger that the attitude of the three masters in November would lead to a domino effect that would see the regional hospitals also halt their plans, and so we decided to talk to the CEOs of the seven hospital groups to see if they could help to maintain the momentum. These, after all, were the people responsible for how the hospitals operated.

It proved difficult to get the CEOs together, and when a teleconference was eventually organized their level of disengagement from the process was dispiriting. They preferred, it seemed, to leave it to individual hospitals to make their own arrangements about providing an abortion service. When pushed, they asked how they should proceed and, somewhat frustrated by this stage, I suggested that 'A plan would be nice.'

Overall it was a disappointing experience, and one that made me question the effectiveness of the group structure as a whole. (Perhaps the six new regional bodies announced in July 2019 to oversee healthcare from 2022 will improve services, although simply giving bodies and people new titles is unlikely to improve their efficacy.)

Another strand of my role was to advise on the details of the legislation passing through the Houses of the Oireachtas. The general outline was well known, having been drafted by the Minister and his Department before the referendum, but it was due to go to Committee for a three-day debate on 6 November. The deadline for submissions of amendments was 31 October. Twenty-four hours before that deadline, ninety-one submissions had been received in total from pro-choice members of the Oireachtas. A Department of Health official told me that she expected a flood of submissions from anti-choice members at the last moment. She was right – another eighty-nine amendments were submitted on the last day, many clearly formulated and timed to slow down the consideration of the legislation.

The draft legislation on the certification process created a difficulty. It was proposed that the same doctor would have to both certify and perform a termination in the less than twelve weeks category. The opinion of the Department was that this was necessary to provide a 'chain of evidence' in the case of litigation. However, given the three-day waiting period, I pointed out that this was not practicable. I gave the example of a consultant seeing a patient on a Wednesday and the woman presenting three days later, on the Saturday, for her termination. The original consultant might be off-duty. It would also be unworkable in GP practices and family planning clinics, where many doctors work part time. The requirement was dropped in the final legislation.

The three-day waiting period itself gave rise to confusion. How should the time be counted? After some discussion the Chief Medical Officer clarified that the clock would have to pass midnight three times; thus if a woman was seen any time on a Monday, for example, she could take the first tablet on the Thursday, provided the pregnancy was still no more than twelve weeks.

In turn, the definition of twelve weeks itself was not straightforward. In obstetric practice a pregnancy is twelve weeks until it is thirteen weeks. Thus twelve weeks and six days is still twelve weeks. However, the Department insisted that the process could not be started later than twelve weeks and zero days (though the termination may not conclude for some days), which meant that a woman had to present at the latest at eleven weeks and three days if she was to fall within the twelve-weeks limit. Interestingly, there was no such insistence on what nine weeks meant.

Towards the middle of December, there was government concern that the majority for passing the legislation in the Seanad was tight. Ironically, the fear was that pro-choice Senators might vote against it because they were unhappy with the three-day waiting period provision (as was I – it was a political compromise, designed to give Tánaiste Simon Coveney cover to support the government's repeal position). The Senators raised the valid concern that, for example, the waiting period might create problems for women in abusive relationships.

On 12 December Dr Mark Murphy and I, together with the Minister, the Chief Medical Officer and other officials met Senators Ivana Bacik, Alice-Mary Higgins, Colette Kelleher, Marie-Louise O'Donnell, Paul Gavan and Lynn Ruane. They were also troubled by the recommendation that a multidisciplinary medical team review cases where a woman's health was at serious risk. It sounded, they thought, like a tri-bunal of inquiry. We were able to reassure them that in fact it is best medical practice to seek the input of appropriate specialists in assessing medical conditions. We answered their various questions as best we could, and the Senators seemed happy with our responses.

Legislation for abortion in Ireland was passed by the Oireachtas and signed into law by President Higgins on 20 December 2018, twelve days before the service was due to start.

There was one last hurdle – the completion of guidelines. The Medi-cal Council had to revise their code of ethics in respect of conscientious objection, while the IOG and ICGP had to prepare comprehensive new guidelines for the service. The draft legislation had been avail-able since early March, and work on guidelines had been under way for several months.

Conscientious objection is well understood and accepted in rela-tion to abortion. Medical Council guidelines are clear: if a doctor has a conscientious objection to treatment, then he or she has a duty to transfer care to another doctor. In an emergency, however, there is no option but to give care. At the Oireachtas Health Committee in Sep-tember, Dr Suzanne Crowe of the Medical Council made it clear that no change in the requirement for referral onwards to another doctor in these guidelines was anticipated when abortion was introduced. (Less well understood, perhaps, is conscientious commitment, i.e., when a doctor is prepared to deliver treatments, giving priority to patient care over adherence to personal religious beliefs or views.)

Technically the revised guidelines could not be formally signed off until the legislation was passed, and any minor final changes in the legislation incorporated. Unfortunately, this did not stop colleagues critical of the 1 January 2019 deadline from complaining publicly in November and December that no guidelines had been issued.

Once the President signed the legislation, the Medical Council and ICGP immediately put forward their guidelines. The IOG simulta-neously circulated completed guidelines where available, and interim guidelines where the work had not been fully completed.

With New Year's Day being a bank holiday, the first patients were not seen until normal working hours resumed on Wednesday,

2 January, and the first GP terminations did not take place until the following weekend.

There were inevitably teething problems, as there are with any new service. This was entirely expected. Indeed, two weeks in advance of the service being launched I told RTÉ Radio One's *This Week* programme that there was 'understandable nervousness about it, and there are a lot of difficulties as we know with infrastructural deficits in the Irish healthcare system'. I also predicted that the service would be 'unrecognizable' after a year.

A week into the operation of the new service, on 8 January, the health correspondent of the *Irish Times*, Paul Cullen, launched an extraordinary broadside under the headline 'A Model of How Not to Bring in a New Service':

The first week of abortion services in Ireland will not go down as a model of good organization, clear communication and open disclosure.

The very opposite: eight days into the new regime, health professionals are still operating with insufficient information and guidance, and little training. The rest of us have been kept in the dark about what services are available, and where.

. . . At most, eight of the State's 19 maternity units were able to provide a service last week. The suspicion is that the actual number of operational units is lower, but the Minister and the HSE have steadfastly refused to provide this information. Nor have they enlightened us on the availability of essential services such as ultrasound or blood testing, or even consultation rooms where women seeking terminations could avail of privacy.

In the community, just 3 per cent of GPs have so far agreed to take referrals from the My Options helpline, and none at all in four counties . . .

What else? Some GPs received training last December 21st – for one day . . .

The legislation hasn't even been published yet online in the normal manner on the Attorney General's website and so is not clearly available as guidance for doctors.

Meanwhile, there was little consultation about the guidelines for the service which, again, were distributed to doctors (but not published) days before the service went live.

These allow a doctor to perform an abortion on a woman aged 15 and under without the involvement of a parent 'in exceptional circumstances'. But what are 'exceptional circumstances' and who makes that decision? Understandably, some doctors feel uncomfortable about the prospect of having to make such a huge ethical decision in the absence of clearer guidelines . . .

The examples of ill-preparation abound. The Medical Council's ethical guidelines have not yet been updated . . .

Of course, many of these problems will be resolved with time. More doctors will sign up; geographical coverage will increase.

Clarity and uniformity will be brought to the provision of services. Problems will be ironed out.

It is also likely, though, that doctors will face uncertainty and difficult ethical decisions because of the rushed manner in which the service was introduced – the very uncertainty the change was supposed to eliminate.

And all because a Minister made a promise he was determined to keep, despite the evidence in front of him.

In a letter to the paper published the next day, I responded in equally robust terms, pointing out that the piece contained some surprising errors and misunderstandings:

Every day since 1 January, people needing to avail of the new service have been successfully using the 24 hour HSE Freephone line and the myoptions.ie website where they have been given appropriate advice and fully informed of what services are available, and where. All those needing to avail of termination services have been accommodated.

At least 200 GPs have signed up to provide the service, with good geographic spread around the country. This is more than enough for the anticipated numbers. Travelling from one county to another is not comparable to the situation before January 1 where people had to leave their own country, alone and at their own expense, to seek treatment that was a criminal offence at home.

The full text of the Health (Regulation of Termination of Pregnancy) Act 2018 is published on the Oireachtas website and is therefore clearly available as guidance for doctors.

Both the Institute of Obstetricians and Gynaecologists (IOG) and the Irish College of General Practitioners (ICGP) have developed and distributed guidelines for doctors. Extensive consultation and research, including travelling to countries that have well established services, was undertaken in the development of these guidelines. Those who need the guidelines have received them.

The article is concerned with what might constitute the 'exceptional circumstances' that might underlie the decision for a young person of 15 or under to seek a termination. One only has to think back to the X case for an understanding of the kind of exceptional circumstances that can occur.

Doctors are faced with ethical decisions very regularly. In such situations both doctors and patients are supported by a range of professionals including social workers and psychiatrists.

Training has been provided since last September for those medical professionals who wished to avail of it and is being provided on an ongoing basis.

It is not the case that the Medical Council Guidelines have not been updated. On December 20 the Council advised all registered doctors on updated revisions which remove 'any conflict between the Ethical Guide and the legislation'. The current guidelines therefore are absolutely clear.

There have been teething problems, as expected, but few that would not have arisen no matter when the service was introduced.

Most of the issues relate to people getting used to a completely new service, and not to lack of preparedness. Each issue that has arisen is being dealt with speedily and comprehensively.

I regret that there are some 'naysayers' willing to spread negativity, some within the medical profession. It is not surprising that medical professionals not currently involved in the provision of termination services have an incomplete and inaccurate understanding of the actual situation.

The *Irish Times* edited out my closing comment, expressing surprise that Paul Cullen – who had my mobile phone number and knew I always responded to his queries – had not contacted me about the piece when writing, despite my role in getting the new abortion service off the ground.

However, I was glad to be able to address what seemed like unfair and one-sided criticisms and let the public know that Irish women had a functioning abortion service, even if we were still ironing out glitches.

Only nine of the nineteen maternity units in the country were listed as providing the service at the beginning of January, and in Dublin the Coombe Hospital wasn't ready until early February. By the end of May, eleven units said they were actively providing the service and all nineteen were dealing with any complications from the community-based service.

Catchment area restrictions imposed early in the year by the Rotunda and the NMH were relaxed when it became apparent that the number of women presenting was less than expected and in keeping with what had been forecast. Indeed, by the end of May, when the eleven units were up and running, the numbers presenting in the under-twelve-weeks category were approximately five per week in the larger hospitals (and fewer in the smaller units).

I find it interesting that the first months of new abortion services have been largely uncontroversial. As I observe the polarized debate in the United States, where provision of services is being rolled back in some states, I can't help but conclude that because abortion was, in effect, imposed on America by a decision of the Supreme Court in 1973, they never had a national debate that looked at the issue in all its complexities. By contrast, in much of Europe, abortion is largely uncontroversial because the law has been made as a result of considerable parliamentary debate.

We await figures on actual numbers for a clear picture of what the first year of legal abortion services in Ireland will look like. As I write this chapter in August, some of the picture is starting to come into focus.

Probably the most salient point is that there have been no complaints from women that they have been unable to access timely, safe abortion services. To me that is reassurance that the service is working well for women. Community provision is clearly working, and indications at the time of writing are that more than 85 per cent, possibly up to 90 per cent, of terminations are happening in the community before nine weeks.

As I have said, planning for the service was based on an expectation of 10,000 terminations per annum. Eight months in, it looks to me as if this figure may be half that, at 5,000 per annum. This is consistent with the numbers who had given an Irish address at UK clinics in recent years and the estimated numbers of those sourcing imported tablets.

As anticipated, the main problem with the service is with the nine-to-twelve-weeks category in the hospitals. The nineteen maternity hospitals and units are severely stretched. These have a consultant staff level that is half the OECD average. The situation with nursing and midwifery numbers is not much better. The impact of staff and funding shortages has pushed gynaecology services to the limit, particularly in those hospitals where the gynaecology unit is integrated into the general hospital.

The ongoing failure of some of the smaller hospitals to provide a service for women with pregnancies complicated by fatal fetal abnormalities is disappointing. It places an unfair burden on the larger hospitals in the hospital groups, which are expected to look after all of the women in the respective regions. In my opinion responsibility for ensuring the service is available in all units is the responsibility of the group CEOs.

In addition to infrastructural shortcomings there are undoubtedly some colleagues who are not willing to provide abortion services. Some of the smaller units have only three or four consultant obstetricians. Where all the consultants have, or say they have, a conscientious objection it is not possible to introduce the service.

In June 2019 the four consultants at St Luke's Hospital in Kilkenny wrote to the chief executive of the Ireland East Hospital Group, Mary Day, and GPs in their area, saying that, following discussions between them, they had 'decided unanimously that the hospital is not an appropriate location for medical or surgical terminations'. They cited a 'multitude of very challenging reasons', though they did not specify these individually. They claimed they did not have a referral pathway into the National Maternity Hospital, the major tertiary referral centre of the Ireland East Hospital Group to which both belong. This is hard to understand, as Kilkenny regularly refers obstetric and gynaecology patients to Holles Street. One of the doctors who wrote this letter was Trevor Hayes, who campaigned against repeal of the Eighth.

A July 2019 investigation by the journalist Ellen Coyne for Joe.ie revealed that this is the case in Letterkenny and Wexford. Also in July Gráinne Ní Aodha reported in TheJournal.ie that correspondence between the National Women and Infants Health Programme and the Department revealed that 'an issue with conscientious objection has prevented the service commencing in Wexford General Hospital.' Wexford said that '[T]here would be an update available in Q2 [May–July [*sic*]] and that there were also "some infrastructural challenges which will need to be addressed".' The refusal by Wexford to provide the service surprised me. When I visited the unit in October 2018, the general manager and the medical staff I met did not see conscientious objection as a major issue and anticipated providing the service in the New Year.

Meanwhile, as Coyne reported, the HSE has stated 'that there were no plans to provide abortion services in South Tipperary General Hospital, because of the low birth rate in the hospital's catchment area and "identified limitations" with resources'. The HSE also said that there were no plans to have abortion services at Portiuncula University Hospital, 'based on a 2018 report into maternity services at the hospital which said that "complex work" at PUH should take place at Galway University Hospital instead'. This is hard to understand, as termination of pregnancy is not a complex procedure.

Ní Aodha's piece reported that Cavan General Hospital had said that it would 'likely be Q3 [August–October [*sic*]] of this year before the hospital "had the staffing to provide the service"'.

In other units, doctors who are providing the service feel isolated and unsupported by colleagues. In early July, Keelin O'Donoghue in Cork wrote in the *Sunday Business Post* that 'Clinical cases can prove divisive among healthcare staff and specialists, which affects working relationships. Doctors like me are being judged by other staff for our views and practice. This is creating conflict in what is an already stressful environment.'

She went on to observe that 'Some healthcare professionals who want to deliver this service feel out of their depth. Many have never worked outside Ireland to see this type of service in practice, but the educational opportunities available to them are limited. Termination of pregnancy represents a huge change in clinical practice, which they see as being forced upon them in a rush.' Her concerns may well be more reflective of local difficulties in Cork than the national situation.

As I write, the HSE now says that ten hospitals of nineteen are providing full abortion services. The Department of Health has made it clear that they want all hospitals to participate. This is a reasonable position. However, if all the consultants in a small unit claim that they conscientiously object to providing the service, there is little the state can do apart from appointing additional consultants who do not object. Attempts are being made in Kilkenny, for example, to do precisely this.

★

I suggest that when information is available about the numbers accessing the service, some of the fears of the hospitals will be allayed. If the most up-to-date estimate of 5,000 terminations per year, with up to 90 per cent being performed in the community, proves correct, then the hospitals will be dealing with very few cases each week – perhaps one or two, or even none some weeks – in the smaller units. It should be possible to set aside one or two clinic appointments per week, and a similar number of operating theatre slots, for a couple of months in order to gauge demand.

To assist clinicians and liaise with hospital managements about providing terminations, it would also be helpful to appoint a clinical lead for the country's abortion service for a couple of years until all the hospitals are on board.

As it turns out, the introduction of abortion services into Ireland has been successful and largely free from controversy. As late as December some were talking about postponing the launch (though by then we had anecdotal reports that bookings by Irish women with UK abortion clinics were down; women were clearly waiting to avail of the local service). My own view was that if we did not at least keep aiming for the deadline, it would drift, and perhaps for months. Deferring the start date was not an option, primarily for political reasons – the Minister had given an undertaking at the end of May and was determined to stick to it (for which he deserves much credit) – but also because women had been assured the service was going to start from 1 January and their expectations could not be dashed. Another month or two might have given everyone involved more time to iron out some of the problems, but no matter when it started there were going to be difficulties. That goes with the territory of setting up any kind of new endeavour.

The fears of some doctors that clinics and operating lists would be swamped have not materialized. Indeed one colleague remarked at an Institute meeting in early January, just a week into the start of the new service, that the women she had treated had been very grateful and she wondered, 'How did we send these patients away before?'

As Nelson Mandela once said, 'It always seems impossible until it's done.'

21. Canon law, St Vincent's and the fate of the National Maternity Hospital

Through most of 2018 the controversy over the relocation of the National Maternity Hospital had receded in the public consciousness. Strangely, not much had happened in the eighteen months since the Religious Sisters of Charity had said they were giving up ownership and management of St Vincent's. There was no move from SVHG to set up the new company to run the hospital. It was mystifying. Approaching the end of the year Holles Street became increasingly concerned about the delay in proceeding with building. New energy requirements – Near-Zero Energy Buildings (NZEB) – were due to come into effect on 1 January 2019, and the NMH fear was that the architectural plans would have to be redesigned and resubmitted to An Bord Pleanála if enabling works on the hospital pharmacy and car park were not commenced before the end of 2018. In December the hospital began a PR blitz to try to move the project on.

Simultaneously, a Campaign against Church Ownership of Women's Health was started and a protest was planned in Dublin for 8 December calling for the NMH to be fully independent. Simon Harris said, '[T]he public was right to believe the Minister should be concerned that the hospital should have "robust governance" and that the State should have a seat at the table when the board was making decisions.'

He said the charitable status of St Vincent's also had to be sorted out, since 'the nuns have said they are leaving' as well as public ownership. The co-leader of the Social Democrats, Deputy Róisín Shortall, was highly critical that a private deal had been done between both hospitals without any regard to the public interest. She asked the Taoiseach to 'consider this – a new public hospital funded by the taxpayer, to be operated by public money and the Minister is pleading for one director on the board to protect the public interest . . . This represents an admission that the Mulvey Report got it completely wrong.'

In early December 2018 the *Irish Catholic* newspaper made a significant contribution to the controversy. It published a story that was the first indication that there were problems afoot in St Vincent's that might explain the lack of movement by SVHG. On Thursday, 6 December, eighteen months after the Sisters of Charity announced their intention to depart, the *Irish Catholic* reported that the Archdiocese of Dublin 'has been left in the dark over plans by the Religious Sisters of Charity to relinquish control of the St Vincent's Healthcare Group and enable the building of a new National Maternity Hospital'. A diocesan spokesperson confirmed that there had been no contact between the sisters and the archdiocese about the issue, 'despite religious orders needing permission from the local ordinary – in the case of St Vincent's, Archbishop Diarmuid Martin – or even the Vatican when seeking to dispose of property above certain values'.* If the NZEB deadline of 1 January was to be met, it would 'not allow for the possibility of the diocese or Holy See vetoing a plan that would entail disposing of Church property to facilitate abortions and other actions contrary to Church teaching'.

The *Irish Catholic* report explained that, under canon law, Irish religious bodies need permission from the local bishop when disposing of assets worth over €348,460. Permission is needed from the Vatican's Congregation for Institutes of Consecrated Life and Societies of Apostolic Life when such assets are valued at more than €3,484,595. The Congregation would typically not approve of such disposals without at least receiving confirmation from the local bishop that he did not object to the religious body's plan. A Dublin diocesan spokesman had earlier confirmed that '[C]anonical requirements are examined only when due process is underway and they cannot be determined in advance.'

Furthermore, a canon lawyer, 'speaking on condition of anonymity', raised the question of whether the sisters had even considered their obligations under Church law when proposing to dispose of the healthcare group, instead seeking only the advice of civil lawyers. 'My experience with civil lawyers is that they don't really understand or even think of canon law. It's very much on the nuns – it's their property, so it's up to them to go through the correct canonical process to alienate. If it goes to Rome, and is not allowed to happen for

---

* Authorship of the report changed in the online edition and for a time it was removed from the website.

immoral purposes, the whole thing could come down on them like a tonne of bricks.'

Despite the statements by Archbishop Martin's spokesperson, Rhona Mahony went on RTÉ's Marian Finucane show on 8 December to argue that it was essential that the Minister for Health agreed to proceeding with the first phase of construction at St Vincent's. This would see funding of €43 million by the state for a new pharmacy and car park at Elm Park. Dr Mahony told Marian Finucane that 'the Sisters of Charity have completely left all elements of SVHG. They have transferred the land, all elements of any involvement they have, into companies, the constitutions of which are with the charities regulator.' She insisted there would be no religious interference 'whatsoever', and that canon law would be 'irrelevant' to its ethos.

As she was speaking, Michael Kelly, editor of the *Irish Catholic*, tweeted: 'Rhona Mahony is quite wrong to say canon law has no role in [the] maternity hospital discussion. The nuns cannot alienate the property without church approval.'

When Marian Finucane put this to Dr Mahony, she replied that 'the Sisters of Charity can take advice but they don't need permission.'

Minutes later Róisín Shortall called the show to question the assertion that the transfer process was complete. When Marian put that to Dr Mahony, she reiterated that the sisters had left all elements of St Vincent's.

The following morning Marian Finucane observed that Rhona Mahony's replies to Michael Kelly and Róisín Shortall had attracted a lot of comment in the Sunday newspapers, and she quoted a spokesperson for the National Maternity Hospital who said, 'We have been told that the constitutions are written and *ready to be submitted* [my italics].' The spokesperson also told RTÉ that on the question of permissions: 'While this is not our issue we understand that the Sisters of Charity have no outstanding requirement for permission or advice from any Church authorities in order to give effect to the decision they announced 18 months ago.'

To be clear, between the two Marian Finucane radio programmes that weekend, Rhona Mahony, and then an NMH spokesperson, had both contradicted the spokesperson for the Archdiocese of Dublin. Crucially, the diocesan spokesperson had signalled the central importance of canon law for the sisters' proposed plan of action. Now, either the diocesan spokesperson was mistaken or the NMH side did not fully grasp what was at stake. Given how things had unfolded up to this point, I had no problem believing that yet again the NMH did not have the full picture.

I told the *Sunday Times* that confirmation by the diocese that there had been no consultation between the Sisters of Charity and it 'has put the whole project in jeopardy. The reported failure to do what they said they would do is a very significant failure. It's a scandal and a tragedy. It is impossible for the government to proceed, unless they want to grant the hospital to the Sisters of Charity. It is clearly unacceptable to transfer the NMH because absolutely nothing has changed.'

I was not altogether surprised when yet another clarification followed from St Vincent's to Sean O'Rourke on the Monday morning. 'We expect the new constitution to be submitted to the Charities Regulator for approval *over the coming weeks* [my italics].' In just forty-eight hours, three separate statements had been made, moving from absolute certainty that the divestment process was already under way to a statement that the paperwork would be submitted some weeks later.

Nicholas Kearns now warned that the entire NMH project would have to return to the drawing board if the contract was not sealed before the new EU regulations came into force at the beginning of 2019, and the Minister for Health was persuaded to approve the first phase of the project; €43 million was made available on 20 December.

Simon Harris announced that agreement had been reached between the Department of Health and St Vincent's regarding protection of the state's interest and the various legal arrangements that were to be put in place regarding changes to the Mulvey agreement, including the appointment of extra directors to the board of the new NMH DAC.

Behind the scenes for the previous year I had been speaking regularly with the Minister and his advisers on the project. I was assured that nothing would be agreed between the Department of Health and the two hospitals until the fully secular St Vincent's charity was established, as promised in May 2017. Despite the failure by St Vincent's to set up the charity, and the confusion issuing from both hospitals as to how far along the process was, I was persuaded by the Minister not to object to the announcement of the new plans. I told him that my continued support was dependent on the new charity being an entirely secular structure, and the public should see evidence of that sooner rather than later. I have repeated this point to him at intervals since. No further development will take place until the ownership structure is in place and has been scrutinized by the Oireachtas and the public.

Nine months later, as this book goes to press, there are still significant questions as to whether St Vincent's are following through on the promises made in May 2017. Construction has been started at Elm Park on the car park and pharmacy, but outside St Vincent's no one has seen the draft constitution of the new secular company.

In June 2019 St Vincent's announced that Rhona Mahony had joined its board. This came as a complete surprise to Holles Street staff and board members. In another rotation of the SVHG board, four new directors had been appointed and three, including the CEO, Professor Michael Keane, retired. A day later, in response to questions on a possible conflict of interests, Nicholas Kearns announced that Dr Mahony had stepped down from the board of Holles Street.

A spokeswoman for St Vincent's told the *Independent* that 'the constitution of the new company, St Vincent's Holdings CLG, was sent to the Companies Registration Office (CRO) for approval in the third quarter of last year [i.e., sometime between July and September 2018].' On 9 June the *Sunday Times* reported that no company of that name could be found on the Companies Registration Office website. I checked again myself in late August. No company of that name was registered at that point. The CRO website states that it takes between five and fifteen working days to register a company.

As for the various statements made to Marian Finucane and Sean O'Rourke in early December 2018, that the constitution of the new St Vincent's company was with the charities regulator, 'ready to go' or would be submitted 'in the coming weeks', Justine McCarthy established in June 2019 that no application had been submitted as of 1 May, some twenty weeks later. It was not until a further fifteen weeks had elapsed that a spokeswoman for the charities regulator confirmed to McCarthy, as she reported on 18 August, that an application had finally been submitted.

★

In writing this book I have come across information that may shine a light on the seemingly inexplicable ongoing delays in making progress with the new St Vincent's company.

From the beginning, I have pointed out that under canon law, Catholic property and its 'charism' – or institutional mission – is subject to the Vatican, unless that property has been alienated by a decision of the Vatican. Alienation, or disposal, of property is covered by canons 1291, 1292, 1293 and 1296.

It is a legal minefield when civil and canon law become entangled, as they have been at St Vincent's. So the Dublin archdiocese's statement to the *Irish Catholic* in December 2018 that there had been no contact between the sisters and the diocese about the issue of alienation of the Elm Park property is more significant than it might at first appear.

It turns out that, behind the scenes, there is major disagreement between the Sisters of Charity and the diocese. I am reliably informed that the sisters are claiming that at some point in the past, they sought and obtained alienation from a previous archbishop of Dublin, and in consequence they now control the property and its use.

The problem for the Sisters of Charity and St Vincent's is that the diocese cannot find evidence of alienation in its records. The sisters have been unable to recall exactly when alienation was granted, or which archbishop granted it, or provide any paperwork to prove their claim. In the absence of any documentation, the Vatican holds the firm view that no alienation has been granted. Therefore, the land belonging to the Sisters of Charity, and its charism, is subject to the Vatican and canon law.

As I have consistently said, as long as any arm of the Catholic Church controls the land, a hospital built at Elm Park must adhere to a Catholic ethos. Given the attention the Vatican is currently paying to events in Ireland, I cannot see how the Vatican will agree to the alienation of the land at Elm Park to permit the construction of a hospital that will perform terminations of pregnancy and other procedures absolutely prohibited by Catholic teaching.

Moreover, in a further difficulty, I have been told that there is no record of the sisters seeking permission from either the diocese or the Vatican to establish St Vincent's Healthcare Group in 2002. This potentially complicates a change of status for the existing SVHG and places a second obstacle in the way of the formation of the so far non-existent St Vincent's Holdings (CLG).

The current archbishop of Dublin, Diarmuid Martin, a man for whom I have great admiration, is on the record as not wishing to have any involvement in Dublin hospitals. However, ultimately he is but a cog in a very large wheel. He is due to retire in mid 2020. It remains to be seen who will be appointed the next archbishop of Dublin.

Meanwhile, the ownership and canon law oversight of the land at Elm Park remains an administrative and legal quagmire that gets deeper and more treacherous as time goes on. I suggest that it would be an act of folly for any Irish government to place confidence in liens or leases granted under civil law while the canon law status of the property remains unresolved and is subject to disagreement between St Vincent's and the Religious Sisters of Charity, the archdiocese of Dublin and the Vatican. Several sets of ambitions – to do with financial interest, legacy-building and the Catholic ethos – are pushing this project. As the delays go on and building inflation rises by 8 per cent or more each month, it is not unreasonable to estimate the final cost of a new national maternity hospital at St Vincent's at €500 million or higher.

One of the reasons I wanted to write this book was to put on the record what I know about the project to locate the National Maternity Hospital on the site of St Vincent's Hospital at Elm Park. The five chapters here are but a summary of a very complicated story. It has been a bruising and stressful experience, but I have no regrets. Having spent my entire professional life working for women's health, I believe it would be a highly retrograde step for the state to sleepwalk into a situation where the flagship maternity hospital of the country adheres to a Catholic ethos. Religious ideology must not harm the women of Ireland any longer.

Epilogue

I knew I was reaching retirement age when a woman accompanying her daughter in childbirth said to me: 'You delivered her twenty-five years ago!' Over the course of my career I estimate that I was present at the birth of, or delivered, more than 6,000 babies. The vast majority were happy events, often affirmed by thank you cards and possibly a bottle or two of wine, though sometimes I received extraordinarily generous presents.*

It is wonderful to meet parents out and about with their children and to see the children growing, and of course to enjoy the wonder in the faces of young children when their mum tells them *He took you out of my tummy*, or to see teenagers squirming when told I was the first person to see them. A woman came up to me at a rugby international in the Aviva Stadium one day to tell me I had delivered her son, who was playing for Ireland that day – a lovely moment, particularly since he was playing in the same position I had played all those years ago.

I enjoyed getting to know some of the fathers who attended antenatal visits. Again, this sometimes led to later encounters in the most unlikely contexts. For instance, one afternoon as I walked towards where my car was parked in Baggot Street, knowing my ticket had probably run out, I could see it being lifted on to a tow truck. The face of the fellow operating the crane fell when he saw me and he said, 'Oh, no, it's not you.' He reversed the crane to deposit my car back on the road, a saving of about €100. Clearly, that birth had gone well.

Despite all of this, the unpredictable nature of obstetrics is one of the most challenging parts of the specialty. A colleague in the US once described it as like a bird flying along happily until it smashes into the windscreen of a jumbo jet it hadn't seen coming. One case illustrates this well. The patient had had an uncomplicated pregnancy, had gone into labour on her due date, and the labour was

---

* A particularly pleasant surprise was the delivery of a case of vintage wine every Christmas for several years!

progressing normally. Because she had an epidural for pain relief, the fetal heart was being continuously electronically monitored and was giving a normal read-out. Suddenly, minutes before birth, the fetal heart stopped. The baby was still-born, and attempts at resuscitation were unsuccessful. A post-mortem examination did not provide any explanation. It was the equivalent of a cot death – sudden and unexpected and with no warning signs. I will never forget my shock at seeing the fetal heart simply stop and the parents' distress at losing their baby so abruptly and inexplicably. Though the vast majority of deliveries go smoothly, events like this never leave you and always hover in the back of your mind.

It was only when I retired from clinical work at the end of 2016 that I realized how much of a presence patients and work had in my mind. I had always thought it essential to retire when performing well and not to hang on for so long that one's skills began to deteriorate – 'to leave the stage while they're still clapping' in other words. Walking out of the labour ward after my last delivery at nine o'clock one mid-December evening, I wondered how I would feel – sad, anxious about the future or happy? I suddenly realized I was, effectively, on holiday for the rest of my life and I could feel the weight lifting from my shoulders. It was only then, and in the following weeks, that I realized how concern about patients was a constant presence in my mind. Had I made the right decision about patient X? Had I missed something in patient Y? Would the outcome have been different if I had done something different for patient Z?

At social occasions non-medics would often ask me how I put up with the unsocial hours and the disrupted sleep. I would compare the job of an obstetrician to someone in a high-powered legal or financial job. Lawyers often have to work late into the night on complicated briefs, only to have the case settle the next morning, and then they have to move on to the next case, an intellectually challenging situation. The person in finance might be asked at short notice, with a family birthday or anniversary imminent, to fly to Japan for an urgent meeting, or to commute to London Monday to Friday on a regular basis, or to be polite at working dinners with people they dislike intensely. The financial rewards might be better, but the lifestyle, and unforgiving nature of the commercial world, did not appeal to me.

The great thing about obstetrics and gynaecology is that it is a very practical, hands-on specialty and you have constant contact with people. Pregnancy is a well-defined process with a clear end: birth. The majority of gynaecological patients have limited duration conditions that are resolved by a well-defined intervention – hysterectomy for example – so there aren't long hours spent poring over complicated documents. Above all, caring for women at the most important times in their lives is a tremendously rewarding way to spend a professional life.

Caring for women was also my motivation for participating in public debate, and particularly for campaigning for the repeal of the Eighth Amendment. On the day I sat in the coroner's court in Galway giving evidence in the case of the tragic and unnecessary death of Savita Halappanavar, it was clear to me that we had reached a crossroads in our attitude to abortion and women's reproductive health. Savita's death had a cathartic effect on Irish society and was the catalyst for an honest conversation about abortion and for changing Irish law for the better. I am very glad to have played a small part in bringing about that change, so that Ireland is a safer and fairer country for women today.

Acknowledgements

I wrote this book over eight months of near-full-time confinement at my desk. Fortunately, Patricia Deevy is a superb editor whose clear vision for the book and wise, informed and acute editorial questions and comments kept me focused on my core objective: to show how some aspects of women's reproductive healthcare in Ireland were out of step with international norms well into the twenty-first century. My experience of working abroad, and my observation of practice at home in Ireland, made me determined to work for change for the better. Patricia's work on the text has enhanced it in so many ways. I am immensely grateful.

Roslyn Dee in Dublin and Donna Poppy in London helped to produce a final manuscript that was clearer, tighter and more polished than I could have achieved.

I am grateful to Michael McLoughlin for commissioning the book and to all at Penguin, especially Aimée Johnston and Orla King. Thanks also to Kieran Kelly for his advice and to Cormac Kinsella for putting me in touch with Michael in the first instance.

Averil Priestman has been my right-hand woman for thirty years and also contributed greatly to the preparation of this book.

As a trainee in St Vincent's and the National Maternity Hospital, I learned from Professor Frank Muldowney the importance of clarity of thought and expression; Mr Frank Duff taught me that every patient should be treated with dignity; and Mr Joe McMullin and Mr Dan Kelly demonstrated an admirable work ethic. At Holles Street, Professor Kieran O'Driscoll, Drs Declan Meagher, Dermot MacDonald and John Stronge were mentors who all, at different stages, facilitated my career progression. All four were masters in sequence, from 1963 to when I started my term in 1991. Drs Carthage Carroll and Malachy Coughlan, who were assistant masters during my time as a junior trainee, were superb colleagues and teachers.

Space does not permit me to thank my medical and midwife colleagues at Holles Street individually, as I would wish, but I am grateful to all. I must, however, mention Maeve Dwyer, who was matron during my mastership, and Mary Brosnan, the current director of midwifery; Cathy Fleming of the antenatal clinics; Margaret Fanagan, who runs antenatal education; Michael Lenehan, who was secretary/manager during my mastership; Brian Davy and Alex Spain, who chaired the executive committee; Kathleen Foley, who warmly welcomed women into the front hall of the hospital; and Betty Hyland and Kay Maguire on the switchboard, who were always welcoming to patients and staff alike who phoned the hospital. Bernadine O'Driscoll was a rock of support during my mastership and beyond.

At Queen Charlotte's and the Chelsea hospitals in London, Sir Jack Dewhurst and Professor Geoffrey Chamberlain provided insights into new ways of dealing with difficult ethical issues in obstetrics. I had many discussions with my trainee colleague Anthony Silverstone, whose reasoned arguments helped to shape my more nuanced views about abortion.

In Houston I learned a huge amount about how to manage change in a department of obstetrics and gynaecology from Bob Creasy. Valerie Parisi and Bernie Gonik, who joined the faculty at the same time as I did, were valued colleagues and friends.

I want to acknowledge the work of medical colleagues who campaigned for repeal of the Eighth Amendment or who have worked on implementation, including Mary Favier, Mary Henry, Veronica O'Keane, Cliona Murphy, Louise Kenny, Mary Higgins, Sabaratnam Arulkumaran, Mary Anglim, Elaine Breslin, Gerry Burke, Nicola Cochrane, Sharon Cooley, Sam Coulter-Smith, Tony Cox, Suzanne Crowe, Sean Daly, Mike Darling (RIP), Jennifer Donnelly, Maeve Eoghan, Chris Fitzpatrick, Rita Galimberti, Richard Greene, Catriona Henchion, John Higgins, Shane Higgins, Trish Horgan, Naro Imcha, Rhona Mahony, Fergal Malone, Brendan McDonnell, Anna McHugh, Peter McParland, Shirley McQuade, Aoife Mullally, Mark Murphy, Meabh Ní Bhuinneain, John O'Brien, Seosamh O'Coighligh, Keelin O'Donoghue, Mike Thompson, Sharon Sheehan, Mary Short and Nóirín Russell.

Many people around the country contributed to the Together for Yes Campaign. I particularly want to thank those I worked with closely, including Deirdre Duffy, Amy Rose Harte, Yvonne Judge, Grainne Griffin, Orla O'Connor, Ailbhe Smyth, Noel Whelan

(RIP), Emma Allen, Christina Sherlock, Lorcan Nyhan and Laura Harmon. Thanks to Bernie Linnane, JoAnne Neary, Lyn Brookes, Tim Spalding, Nora Newell, Alan McMenamin and Sharon McMenamin in Leitrim and Donegal. The Termination for Medical Reasons group, and those women who described their own abortion experiences, deserve enormous credit for their courage in coming forward.

Many other individuals and organizations have contributed to the advocation and implementation of change, including Niall Behan of the IFPA, Alison Begas and Shirley McQuade of the Well Woman Centre, Fintan Foy and Helen McVeigh of the ICGP, and Dr Gavin Briggs and Barry Downes of Affidea.

Leo Kearns, Barbara Conneely and Stephanie Good of the IOG, provided essential support both during my tenure as chair of the IOG and during preparations for implementation of the termination of pregnancy service. Thanks also to Ruth Sliedrecht of PwC.

At the Department of Health and HSE, Geraldine Luddy, Tony Holohan, Eamonn Quinn, Kilian McGrane, Aisling Heffernan, Peter McKenna, Dean Sullivan, David Hanlon, Angela Dunne, Sheila Sugrue, John Hennessy, Pat Healy, Kate Mulvenna, Sally Downing, Sarah Hamza and Pheena Kenny all played important roles in effecting change.

I have always found Simon Harris, Minister for Health, receptive to advice and found his commitment to change admirable. Interactions with the various politicians involved in the campaign gave me a new respect for how politics can effect change when there is common purpose, commitment and cross-party cooperation. I would like to thank particularly An Taoiseach Leo Varadkar, Senator Catherine Noone, Senator Jerry Buttimer, Senator Ivana Bacik, Deputy Róisín Shortall, Deputy Alan Kelly, Deputy Charlie Flanagan, Senator Lynn Ruane, Councillor Brendan Carr and Councillor Mícheál Mac Donncha.

I have quoted extensively from contemporaneous newspaper reports and opinion pieces. For reasons of space and clarity, and because the articles are mainly searchable online, I have not referenced each one. However, I am indebted to the work of the following journalists and commentators whose work has informed the text: Justine McCarthy, Colin Coyle, *Sunday Times*; Patsy McGarry, Kitty Holland, Paul Cullen, Martin Wall, Sarah Bardon, Mary Minihan, Jack Power,

Sarah Burns, Ronan McGreevy, Pat Leahy, Fiach Kelly, John McManus, Michael O'Regan, Fintan O'Toole, Vivienne Clarke, Harry McGee, Una Mullally, Kathy Sheridan and Marie O'Halloran, *Irish Times*; Eilish O'Regan, Dearbhail McDonald, Kevin Doyle, Philip Ryan, Cormac McQuinn, Maeve Sheehan, Jody Corcoran, Eoin O'Malley, *Irish Independent* and *Sunday Independent*; Neil Michael, Leah McDonald, Katie O'Neill, Senan Molony, Jennifer Bray, Darren Hassett, John Lee, Philip Nolan, Eithne Tynan, *Irish Daily Mail*; Fiachra Ó Cionnaith, Jimmy Woulfe, Catherine Shanahan, Dan Buckley, Fergus Finlay, *The Examiner*; Susan Mitchell, Róisín Burke, Mary Regan, Michael Brennan, Hugh O'Connell, Susan O'Keeffe, *Sunday Business Post*; Ellen Coyne, Catherine Sanz, *The Times (Ireland)*; Ger Colleran, *The Star*; Priscilla Lynch, June Shannon, Catherine Reilly, *Irish Medical Independent*; Gary Culliton, *Irish Medical News*; Lloyd Mudiwa, *Irish Medical Times*; Michael Kelly, Greg Daly, *Irish Catholic*; and Henry McDonald, *Guardian*.

I am grateful to Professor Noel Whelan, former chairman of St Vincent's Healthcare Group for twenty-six years, Michael Somers, and my late father-in-law, Don Mahony, deputy chairman of the board of the Mater Hospital, who provided much valuable background to interactions between hospitals, the state and the Catholic Church.

My sister Anna Farmar has been a valuable source of advice both throughout my life and during the writing of this book. Her late husband Tony's work *Holles Street 1894–1994* provided me with much useful information about the hospital.

Finally, my wife Jane was a rock of support, offering constructive criticism throughout. She acted as a sounding board at every stage and undertook an immense amount of background research. Her experience as an academic publisher was of great value in helping me to understand the process of writing a book. I am eternally grateful.

Index